The Healing Power *of* Fever

The
Healing Power
of
Fever

Your Body's Natural Defense against Disease

Christopher Vasey, N.D.

Translated by Jon E. Graham

Healing Arts Press
Rochester, Vermont • Toronto, Canada

Healing Arts Press
One Park Street
Rochester, Vermont 05767
www.HealingArtsPress.com

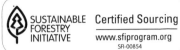

SUSTAINABLE FORESTRY INITIATIVE   Certified Sourcing
www.sfiprogram.org
SFI-00854

Text stock is SFI certified

Healing Arts Press is a division of Inner Traditions International

Originally published in French under the title *La fièvre, une amie à respecter* by Éditions Jouvence, S.A., Chemin du Guillon 20, Case 143, CH-1233 Genève-Bernex, Switzerland, www.editions-jouvence.com, info@editions-jouvence.com
First U.S. edition published in 2012 by Healing Arts Press

Note to the reader: This book is intended as an informational guide. The remedies, approaches, and techniques described herein are meant to supplement, and not to be a substitute for, professional medical care or treatment. They should not be used to treat a serious ailment without prior consultation with a qualified health care professional.

Library of Congress Cataloging-in-Publication Data

Vasey, Christopher.
  [Fièvre, une amie à respecter. English]
  The healing power of fever : your body's natural defense against disease / Christopher Vasey ; translated by Jon E. Graham. — 1st U.S. ed.
      p. cm.
  Summary: "A guide to the healing and detoxifying effects of fever"— Provided by publisher.
  Includes index.
  ISBN 978-1-59477-437-9 (pbk.) — ISBN 978-1-59477-799-8 (e-book)
  1. Fever therapy. 2. Alternative medicine. I. Title.
  RM868.V3713 2012
  615.5—dc23
                                                                2011038500

Printed and bound in the United States by Lake Book Manufacturing
The text stock is SFI certified. The Sustainable Forestry Initiative® program promotes sustainable forest management.

10 9 8 7 6 5 4 3 2 1

Text design by Viginia Scott Bowman and layout by Priscilla Baker
This book was typeset in Garmond Premier Pro, with Helvetica Neue and Agenda used as display typefaces

To send correspondence to the author of this book, mail a first-class letter to the author c/o Inner Traditions • Bear & Company, One Park Street, Rochester, VT 05767, and we will forward the communication, or visit the author's website at **www.christophervasey.ch/EN/HOME.html**.

Contents

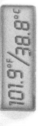

Introduction

As a general rule fever is considered something bad that needs to be fought. In reality it is the result of the effort made by the body to defend itself against an infection or a poison.

Fever is the expression of this protective work. The intensified functioning of the various organ systems involved in the defense response heats up the body, hence the rise in temperature. Striving to eliminate a fever amounts to opposing the body's natural defense mechanisms; in other words, countering the healing efforts that are implemented as nature intended.

This book explains just what fever is and how to assess its various manifestations and the different stages through which it passes. It also describes how to maintain a fever to achieve true healing and how to control a fever when it becomes too fierce. The techniques provided are simple, natural, and accessible to everyone. They are all based on a commonsense approach and include procedures for treatment based on diet, hydrotherapy, and the use of medicinal herbs.

The majority of fevers are caused by infection. This book will not discuss anti-germ strategies, however. The use of natural antibiotics is a subject in its own right, which I covered in great detail in my book on natural alternatives to antibiotics.*

The advice offered in this book for treating a fever should not be regarded as a substitute for the care and follow-up treatment of a trained health professional. Some fevers can conceal dangerous infections that the overeating, stressed out humans of the twenty-first century, whose bodies are weakened by regular exposure to toxins and pollutants, cannot vanquish all on their own. Stronger measures will sometimes be called for. Good common sense should always be used: anything that cannot be easily mastered should be left to the care of a professional.

This book will also describe how to create an artificial fever as a means of treating the body in advance. In other words, we can employ fever as a preventive tool to renew the cellular terrain of the body before the toxins stagnating there can trigger any kind of disease. This book therefore addresses both readers who are sick and seeking care as well as those who are healthy and wish to remain so.

---

*Christopher Vasey, *Alternatives naturelles aux antibiotiques* (Genève-Bernex, Switzerland: Éditions Jouvence, 2004).

Part One

Understanding
Fever

Most people think of fever only as the unpleasant period of time during which the body's temperature is too high. But to those who understand its different manifestations, fever reveals the intensity with which the body fights against illness. When we understand how this mechanism is working against infection, we can derive useful hints on how to support these efforts. Fever is one of the most powerful defenses of the body. For optimal health, it is essential to have an understanding of its characteristics.

1

The Temperature of the Human Body

Before studying the characteristics of fever, it is important to first have an understanding of how the body regulates its temperature.

HOMEOTHERMIA

Humans are *homeothermic*, which means that their body temperature should always remain the same with almost unvarying consistency. In other words, it does not change in accordance with the weather or with atmospheric conditions. Whether it is summer or winter, whether people live in the desert or the far

north, their body temperature will always stay around
98.6°F. This is the core temperature (inside the body)
and not the more superficial reading of 97.7°F provided by taking the temperature with a thermometer
placed beneath the arm. In the animal kingdom the
other homeotherms are mammals such as goats and
cows and so forth, as well as birds.

The word *homeotherm* is used to describe the
opposite of the *poikilotherm*. Poikilothermic animals'
body temperature varies in accordance with the ambient temperature of their environment. The temperature
of these animals will rise when the sun is shining and
the weather is hot, such as during the summer, for
example, and will fall when it is cloudy, during the
night, and during the cold seasons of the year.

One well known example can be used to illustrate
these variations of body temperature in response to
climatic condition: the lizard. When stretched over a
stone, basking in the sun, its body temperature can
rise higher than 104°F. During colder periods of the
year, the lizard's temperature can fall to 68°F, 50°F,
or even 41°F, depending on the temperature of its
environment. Given that the speed of its metabolism
is dependent on its internal heat, in summer the lizard
can flee with lightning speed, but when the weather
turns cold it moves so slowly that it can be trapped
without any difficulty.

Some animals, such as hibernating mammals, combine both systems: they are homeotherms in the spring and summer, but with the arrival of winter they fall into the slumber of hibernation and their body temperature matches that of their environment.

It was once common to make a distinction between warm-blooded and cold-blooded animals, but this terminology has been abandoned since the lizard, for example, theoretically a cold-blooded animal, can have a body temperature much higher than we humans who are technically warm-blooded beings!

The fact that they are capable of producing the heat necessary to maintain a consistent body temperature gives homeotherms—therefore human beings—a remarkable kind of freedom and independence. No matter what the conditions outside might be, homeothermic beings are able to move about, take care of their daily business, and defend themselves against danger.

While there are numerous advantages to being a homeotherm, there are also several drawbacks. First and foremost, homeotherms can tolerate only minimal variations in body temperature. At several degrees higher than the norm, up to 109.4°F to be exact, the mechanisms sustaining life in the body will be destroyed thus bringing on death. When the core temperature drops several degrees below the norm, to 86°F, in fact, vital functions will be paralyzed, also causing death.

HEAT IS NECESSARY
FOR LIFE

The ideal temperature for the functioning of the human body is 98.6°F. This is the temperature required for the enzymes to diligently perform all the biochemical transformations necessary to organic life. Just like the chemist in the laboratory will heat the test tube when trying to combine two substances that are non-miscible in the ambient conditions, the body needs a certain degree of heat in order to function. Countless chemical substances need to be transformed, combined, separated, and recycled in the body for energy production to take place, as well as the building and repair of tissue, respiration, digestion, and so forth. The temperature of 98.6°F is also necessary for the organs to function at their optimum levels. Thanks to heat, our bodies are able to function, and, by functioning, our bodies produce the heat that helps them perform all their activities.

Because our body temperature is always stable, and without any effort required on our behalf to consciously maintain it, we often do not realize just how important it is. Yet heat is always associated with life and the living and cold is forever associated with death. A certain internal heat is essential for our survival.

THE BODY'S PRODUCTION OF HEAT

Body heat is produced in multiple ways. Let's begin by looking at the most obvious ways: physical activity and digestion.

The contraction of muscles releases heat; for, like all machines, whether a car or a washing machine, the rubbing of different parts against one another produces heat. Added to this heat production is that of the "combustion" of sugars in the muscles. By combustion I mean the transformation of sugar into energy that can be utilized by the muscles. This is how any physical activity—walking, carrying, working, speaking—can produce heat.

The digestive process also provides heat to the body. On the one hand this is because an entire series of organs—the stomach, liver, pancreas, and intestines—is working and therefore releasing heat. On the other hand it is because the foods that are eaten also supply it. Their constituent substances are "burned" by the body and transformed into caloric energy. Foods that are cooked and eaten while still warm will provide additional heat to the body.

Even in the absence of movement and digestion, such as at night when we are sleeping, our bodies continue to produce heat. This heat comes from the billions of cells making up our functioning organism. Vital functions such as breathing and blood circulation have to be maintained without stop in order to keep the body alive, even if they are taking place at a slower pace. This minimal activity (life could not be sustained at a lower rate) is what we call the basic metabolism.

Respiration contributes to the production of heat inasmuch as the ceaseless movements of inhalation and exhalation within the rib cage are triggered by the work of the different muscles.

Blood circulation occurs thanks to the beating of the heart, which provides an uninterrupted source of heat for the body. When one part of the heart contracts to propel blood into the vessels, the other part is working to aspirate blood toward the heart. In addition to these heat sources is the friction of the blood as it travels along the walls of the vessels and that of the air in the respiratory tract. Both of these frictions produce heat. Their level of heat production becomes even more considerable when their speed of movement is increased, for example, because of sustained physical activity.

The heat produced by the basic metabolism is added to that produced by the other organs and that generated by the muscles during physical exercise or by the digestive tract when we are eating. The allocation of this heat is then governed by the blood, which, thanks to its incessant circulatory movement, transports this heat produced in each specific organ throughout the body.

HEAT LOSS

Opposing this constant production of heat is the loss of that heat. This is a permanently occurring situation by virtue of the fact that human beings live in environments that are most often cooler than the average temperature of the human body.

In the temperate zones of the earth, the average temperature outside is 77°F in the summer and 40°F during the winter, therefore varying from around 21 to 56 degrees cooler than that of our bodies. Even inside our houses the temperature is cooler, most thermostats being set between 68°F and 72°F.

It is thus inevitable for our bodies to lose heat because of environmental circumstances even though we dress more or less warmly depending on the season. This expression "warmly" is not entirely accurate since the clothing is not producing any heat, it is preventing heat from leaving the body.

In order for a naked human body to avoid losing heat to the ambient environment, the temperature should be around 89°F to 90°F. This is rarely the case and when it does occur is only temporary. So, as a rule, we are in a situation of losing heat on a constant basis.

REGULATION OF TEMPERATURE

When there is too much heat loss, the body has a variety of steps it can take for quickly correcting the problem.

One of the body's short-term measures for producing heat involves collecting the heat created on the body's surface through the contraction of muscles called the *arrectores pilorum* (the hair erector muscles). Although quite small, these muscles are large in quantity and can produce a measureable amount of heat on the skin surface. Their contraction creates the effect we know as goose bumps. Shivering, shaking limbs, and chattering teeth are all additional defense system reactions for confronting cold conditions. They contribute to the maintenance of body temperature through the heat they produce.

These measures are superficial, though, and aid from a deeper defense system must also be called upon. This consists of the body's acceleration of its metabolism. By intensifying the cardiac rhythm and the amplitude of respiration, combustions increase and increased heat is supplied to the body. This metabolic acceleration is achieved by means of the nervous and hormonal systems, the thyroid and adrenal glands in particular. It can be set in motion at any time and its intensity regulated based on the body's needs. The major director of these operations is the hypothalamus.

While it is easy for the body to intensify its metabolic activities to combat the cold, it is not, in contrast, so easy for it to reduce them to protect itself from excessive heat. In fact, it is impossible for the body to slow organic activity any lower than the basic metabolism rate that is essential for the body's survival.

Because the body has no efficient means for reducing its naturally occurring production of heat, its one remaining option is to increase the amount of heat that the body naturally loses. It manages this through cutaneous vasodilation. By dilating the blood vessels at the surface of the skin and bringing more blood charged with this excess heat from the depths of the body to the periphery, the body encourages heat loss. An increase in pulmonary ventilation (breathing) will also achieve this goal. The intensification of respiratory movements makes it possible to expel a larger volume of heat-charged air and to inhale a larger quantity of fresh air, which will cool the body. This process is especially visible in dogs who will pant with their mouths wide open and their tongues hanging out when they are too hot. Dogs, in fact, hardly sweat and have to regulate their body temperature through their respiratory tracts.

Mentioning sweat leads naturally to the third means the body has for eliminating excess heat. Through evaporation, the small drops of sweat secreted by the sudoriferous (sweat) glands cool down the skin. In fact, in order to evaporate, these drops have to remove heat from the body. The more one perspires, the more this perspiration evaporates and the greater the amount of heat removed from the body.

CORE TEMPERATURE AND
PERIPHERAL TEMPERATURE

Saying that the body's temperature is 98.6°F can give the impression that this temperature is uniform throughout the entire body. However, this is not possible; there are necessarily some regions that are less hot than others.

The cooler regions of the body are those that are in contact with the outside, where the loss of heat caused by the body's contact with a colder environment takes place. The hottest region of the body is where the heat-producing organs are located, which is to say, inside the body. The temperature of this region remains constant because this part of the body is surrounded and protected by the body's surface layers. The temperature of the outer portions of the body will change slightly depending on the conditions of the outside environment.

The temperature of 98.6°F that has been designated as that of the human body is that of the interior of the human body taken as a whole. (Some organs, the liver, for example, have a higher temperature.) For this reason, this temperature is also called the *core* temperature, in contrast to the *peripheral* temperature of the body's outer layer.

The core of the human body consists of:

- The brain
- Internal organs of the torso such as the stomach,

liver, spleen, pancreas, lungs, kidneys, heart, and blood vessels
• The central portions of the arms and legs

It should be emphasized that the closer one moves toward the limbs' extremities, the smaller the core zone becomes, eventually vanishing completely in the hands and feet. The peripheral zone of the body, in which the temperature may vary, consists of the skin and the tissue lying directly under it. This zone is therefore quite thin but since it covers the entire body it still represents a large mass.

The temperature of the body's peripheral layer varies as a result of two factors: the volume of the core zone it surrounds and the outside temperature. When the outside temperature is, for example, 68°F, the peripheral temperature will be 96.8°F at the level of the torso but will fall to 93.2°F and 89.6°F respectively at the thighs and biceps and 87.8°F and 82.4°F at the shinbones and forearms (see figure 1b on page 16).

If the outside temperature falls to 32°F, the temperature of the body's peripheral layers will continue to fall but not beyond a certain physiological limit. Protective mechanisms in the body will work to keep the temperature up and preserve life in the tissue. In contrast, when the outside temperature climbs higher, to 104°F, for example, the core zone will increase, extending all the way out to the periphery instead of stopping a certain distance away (see figure 1c on page 16).

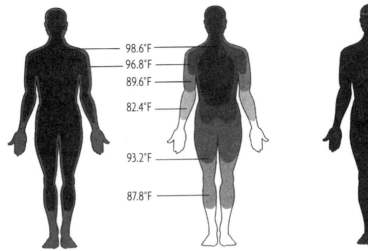

a) Exposure to an external temperature of 96.8°F shows the core zone clearly distinguished from the peripheral zone.

b) Exposure to an external temperature of 68°F shows a further reduction of the core zone.

c) Exposure to heat or fever (104°F); expansion of the core zone out to the periphery.

Figure 1. Variations of internal temperature based on the outside environment (according to Jürgen Aschoff; adapted from his own illustration)

MEASURING BODY TEMPERATURE

The measure of a patient's body temperature with a thermometer allows the caregiver to verify if he or she is "running a high temperature," in other words a fever, and how high it is. Fever, to put it plainly, occurs anytime the body's temperature is higher than its normal state. By taking repeated readings over the course of the day, the caregiver can follow the fever's evolution and determine whether it is rising or falling.

There are two kinds of thermometers commonly available. The most simple, and completely effective nonetheless, consists of a graduated tube containing liquid. Formerly this liquid was always mercury. Today, for safety reasons, as mercury is highly toxic, it has been replaced by colored alcohol. With this type of thermometer, after the temperature reading has been taken you must shake the tube to make the liquid fall back to the bottom and be ready for the next reading. The more recent kind of thermometer is electronic; it works on batteries and has a flexible mouthpiece. A digital screen indicates the body temperature to the nearest fraction.

As discussed previously, the core temperature of the human body (98.6°F) is not identical to that of the more superficial zones that can be reached by the standard thermometer. The temperature will be slightly cooler when the reading is taken close to the surface of the body. The body's normal temperature when measured on the surface is 97.7°F and the onset of fever is marked as 98.6°F* although this is a perfectly normal temperature for the core zone.

There are a number of natural cavities on the body where the temperature can be taken with a thermometer. The armpit, mouth, rectum, and inner ear cavities allow you to get beyond the surface of the body. These

---

*On nondigital thermometers this point is generally highlighted in red.

areas are also in the proximity of significant blood vessels, which transport blood of the same temperature as the core zone.

The axillary (armpit) temperature reading is the most commonly used as it is the easiest to execute. It is not as intrusive as the other options, and it is suitable for every age group except that of small children and infants. The thermometer should be placed in the base of the armpit with the arm closed around it so that the tip of the thermometer is completely enveloped, which will bring the temperature reading closer to that of the body's core temperature. The normal temperature of this area is between 96.6°F and 98°F.

An oral temperature reading is obtained by placing the head of the thermometer in the mouth at the back of the cavity found beneath the tongue. The patient must keep his mouth closed and avoid drinking or eating anything hot for the half hour preceding the temperature reading. This method is rarely usable for infants but is perfectly suitable for older children and adults. The normal temperature for this area is between 97.8°F and 98.4°F.

A rectal temperature reading is much closer to that of the core temperature, because the measurement is taken at a deeper level in the body. The thermometer should be inserted 2 to 3 centimeters into the rectum. The use of a lubricating agent is recommended. It is essential to use an unbreakable thermometer here or one with a flexible tip, especially when this method is used on babies. The normal temperature in this area is between 98.4°F and 99.1°F. Because of the more invasive nature of this procedure, it is no longer one of the most commonly used methods.

Ear temperature is almost identical to the body's core temperature. A large vessel from deep within the body passes in close proximity to the tympanic membrane (eardrum) carrying blood to this area directly from the center of the body. The eardrum is also close to the hypothalamus, the major regulating center of body temperature. To take a person's temperature in the ear, you must use a special thermometer designed specifically for this purpose, and it must be placed exactly on the eardrum and not on the walls of the ear canal.

Locations for Taking Thermometer Readings

- Armpit
- Mouth (beneath the tongue)
- Rectum
- Ear (on the eardrum)

During the course of a fever, the temperature should always be taken with the same thermometer, at the same spot, and at the same times in order for useful comparisons to be made. It is a good idea to take the temperature three times a day: once in the morning upon waking, once in the afternoon around 2 p.m. (before or after an afternoon nap), and once in the evening around 7 or 8 p.m. This final measurement is often the most revealing. Furthermore, it is helpful to know that fever often climbs after 5 p.m. In order to better monitor the evolution of the illness, it is sometimes necessary to take one or two additional readings. Doing so enables the caregiver to better interpret the changes in the patient's condition.

Summary

The ideal temperature for the human body, the one that allows biochemical transformations to occur without problem and for optimum organ function, is 98.6°F. The body works continuously to maintain this temperature.

2

Natural Variations in Temperature

Although the core temperature of 98.6°F is presented as a stable value, it can vary slightly depending on various factors.

On waking up from a full night's sleep, the core temperature is around 97.7°F. This is a bit lower than the temperature of the body for most of the day, which is explained by the fact that the body functions at a slower rate during the night. At the end of the day, the opposite is true, and the temperature is slightly higher at 99.5°F. This is because the body has collected heat generated by its physical activities over the course of the day. This means there is a normal deviation of almost a degree on either side of the optimum temperature of 98.6°F. This is a minimal distinction, but larger deviations are possible.

When temperature deviations are evident on the low end of the scale, with body temperatures around 96.8°F and even as low as 95°F on a daily basis, it can indicate a state of permanent hypothermia. These are people whose vitality has been greatly diminished following a long illness, a protracted and exhausting activity, long periods of hardship and deprivation, or with age or certain diseases such as cardiac disorders, which reduce the oxygenation of the tissues and consequently reduce the intensity of the metabolism in general.

The core temperature cannot fall much lower than this without serious consequence; 86°F qualifies as life-threatening, severe hypothermia, with symptoms such as loss of muscle coordination and even loss of consciousness. In exceptional cases, individuals whose body temperatures have fallen as low as 68°F following prolonged exposure to the cold—boating accident victims and mountain climbers—have been saved and brought back to health. But these are very rare cases.

Nonetheless, in certain surgical procedures the body temperature is intentionally brought to the critical 86°F mark for a brief period of time in order to slow blood circulation and metabolic activities. The temperature of a single organ may be brought down even further during certain operations, sometimes as low as 50°F; this is therefore localized hypothermia and not a general case.

Temperature deviations upward (*hyperthermia*) are also possible, but the body is unable to tolerate as much upward deviation. A rise of several degrees and the body reaches its upper limit of 109.4°F, after which death ensues.

NATURAL AND PATHOLOGICAL HYPERTHERMIA

Naturally occurring hyperthermia is the result of intensified physical activity. For workouts and sporting activities, a temperature between 101.3°F and 102.2°F is considered optimum for the flexibility of the muscles and tendons. The core temperature can rise as high as 104°F with strenuous activity, which is not optimum but still acceptable.

A large production of heat and an increase in body temperature will also occur during a large meal accompanied by alcohol, as this makes a great demand on the forces of the body. It is common to see diners who are flushed and even perspiring.

Sauna is another practice that causes a rise in body temperature. Enveloped in air that often ranges between 176°F and 212°F causes the body to collect large amounts of heat without the possibility of losing very much of it. Adding this heat to the existing body heat induces hyperthermia.

A common characteristic of these different forms of hyperthermia is that they are only temporary and do not last for long periods of time. After a maximum of several hours after the activity has ceased, the optimum temperature of 98.6°F will return.

The same cannot be said for hyperthermia of pathological origin, in other words, fevers. Fevers, with their characteristic ups and downs, do extend over longer periods of time, and can last for several days or weeks.

FEVER

Strictly speaking, we are dealing with fever when—because of an illness—the body's core temperature rises more than 1.8 degrees above its normal temperature.

When the temperature range falls between 99.5°F and 100.4°F, we are dealing with a sub-feverish condition or febricule. The onset of genuine fever is defined as starting at 100.4°F. Fever is more or less intense depending on how much higher than normal body temperature it has become. Temperature in the range from 100.6°F to 101.3°F is described as mild fever. Higher than this, up to 102.2°F is moderate fever. A strong fever is a temperature of 102.3°F or higher, and a severe fever is 104°F or higher. While fever spikes of between 105.8°F and 107.6°F can be tolerated, anything over 109.4°F will be fatal.

Fever Classifications

Mild fever: 100.6°F to 101.3°F

Moderate fever: 101.4°F to 102.2°F

Strong fever: 102.3°F to 103.9°F

Severe fever: 104°F and higher

During a fever, the temperature of the peripheral layer of the body is the same as the core temperature; whereas, under normal conditions it is always slightly lower. With the core temperature of the body extending all the way to the surface, the entire body is bathed in an intense heat, which it can barely tolerate—especially when the temperature is quite high and lasts for extended periods of time (see figure, page 16).

These high temperatures bring about functional disorders, with disruption of enzymatic activity, blood circulation, cellular exchanges, nerve transmission, and muscular contractions. If severe fever continues, the heat will cause the macro-proteins of the body organs to break down, forming lesions. The lesions will not allow the organs to function properly, and death will soon follow.

THE CAUSES OF FEVER

There are numerous causes of fever, the best known being microbial infection. The bacteria, viruses, funguses, and parasites that are able to find a way into our bodies are the source of many diseases. Poisoning, allergic reactions, and the presence of cancerous cells are additional causes of fever. Overeating and physical exhaustion are also common culprits.

What do these various causes have in common? Germs, poisons, allergens, toxins, and so forth all threaten the proper functioning of the body and its very survival. All of these substances and conditions, diverse as they may be, oblige the body to react in order to protect itself from their harmful influence. The reaction of physiological defenses consists first and foremost of neutralizing and eliminating anything that represents a danger.

Microbes themselves are a danger because they destroy whatever tissue they colonize. Because they are living beings, they also expel excrement into our bodies. Their waste products overwhelm the body either because of the mass they represent—although germs are tiny, during an infection they quickly multiply and become numerous—or because of their toxicity. Some of these germs are true poisons for our cells; for example, the toxins of *Clostridium tetani,* which are responsible for tetanus and which destroy the nerve cells of the spinal column and muscles.

The mineral, plant, and animal substances responsible for poisoning people, like caustic soda, for example, or mushroom toxins or snake venom, are harmful to the body by definition because they either disrupt its proper functioning or attack its tissues. Allergens are dangerous because of their specific characteristics and the wide range of physiological and chemical reactions they cause; cancerous cells release dangerous poisons; overeating creates massive amounts of metabolic residues and wastes; and mental and physical overexertion, too, threaten health because of the wastes they produce, which cannot be eliminated by the body in a timely manner.

Fever is therefore not a symptom that is imported by the poison or germs but the expression of the body as it confronts this attack. Fever is not an independent entity that comes from the outside; it develops in response to an external threat. This explains why fever is present in so many different kinds of diseases and disorders.

To really understand how the body "makes" a fever, we must first take a good look at a fundamental notion of natural medicine, that of the biological terrain.

THE BIOLOGICAL TERRAIN

The body will be able to function properly, which is to say, enjoy good health, only if its organs are working normally. These organs can work well only if the cells they consist of are able to faithfully perform their duties. This capability depends entirely on the organic fluids in which the cells are immersed.

The cells are entirely dependent upon these fluids: they are the source of their nutrition, the means for transporting their wastes away, and their medium for transferring information. In fact, cells are entirely surrounded—inside and out—by fluid. This vast ocean in which they live consists of blood, extracellular fluid (which surrounds the cells), and intracellular fluid (with which they are filled). All together, these liquids make up what is known as the biological terrain—the internal cellular environment of the body. And just as a plant can thrive only in soil or a terrain possessing very specific properties, cells can live only in a suitable biological terrain.

There is an ideal composition of these bodily fluids that allows the body to function at its optimum level. Consequently, the balance of health is threatened by each and every qualitative change of this composition. Two principal alterations may occur:

- either the fluids lack certain substances (vitamins, minerals, and so forth) needed to achieve and maintain their ideal composition,
- or the terrain is overloaded with substances that should not be there (toxins, poisons, pollutants, contaminants) or should not be there in such large quantity (metabolic residues and wastes such as urea, uric acid, other acids, and cholesterol).

In the first case, we are dealing with deficiencies; in the second case, the clogging and fouling of the terrain by toxins. This clogged and fouled state of the terrain is regarded in natural medicine as the primary cause of disease.

These wastes can irritate the cells causing inflammation or sclerosis, or they can obstruct and smother them. They make the blood thicker, clog blood vessels, and cause congestion in the organs. They disrupt cellular exchanges. The basic problem of ill health is found first in the biological terrain. It becomes visible on the "surface" only later when dysfunction becomes apparent in one part of the body or another.

ILLNESS:
A DEFENSIVE REACTION

The body does not remain a passive spectator to the invasion of its tissues by wastes and poisons. It reacts and seeks to rid itself of them by either eliminating them from the body or by burning them on site.

Eliminations take place thanks to the excretory organs, which filter wastes from the blood and lymph and then expel them from the body. These organs include the respiratory tract, skin, liver, intestines, and kidneys. The eliminations that result from the increased labor of these organs are exhibited in catarrhs affecting the respiratory tract (runny nose or sinus, expectorations);

eruptions on the skin (pimples, acne, eczema); diarrhea, vomiting, or bile attacks; increased urination and urine that is thick, acidic, irritating, and dark.

The second means the body has at its disposal for ridding itself of wastes is to "burn" them, breaking them down into smaller particles that will be easier to eliminate. These combustions are achieved through increased oxygen intake and increased enzymatic activity. In turn, this necessitates and triggers an accelerated rate of exchanges and an increased speed of blood circulation and respiratory rhythm. The overall intensification of the metabolism engenders an increase in body temperature, in other words, this causes a fever.

WHAT HAPPENS DURING A FEVER?

What happens during a fever, when the body defends itself against an attack? Let's first take the case of a fever caused by microbial infection before we look at those caused by poisons or toxins.

As soon as the immune system detects an infection, it activates the body's natural defenses. This automatically causes an acceleration of blood flow through the vessels and, consequently, also increases the heart rate. The acceleration of blood circulation ensures the rapid transport of the body's defenders from the place they are produced to the site of infection. There is little use in having an army of soldiers if they are not on the battlefield.

Among these defenders that have to be transported are the macrophages, large cells that destroy germs by swallowing them whole, later digesting them in a process known as *phagocytosis*. Macrophages normally reside in the tissues. In the event of an infection, they have to travel through the extracellular fluid and lymph to reach the site of the infection, whereupon they can spring into action. Microphages are smaller in size but act in the same manner. They primarily reside in the blood. The blood flow carries them to the site of the infection where they leave the vessels and enter the affected tissues in order to absorb the germs that they find there.

T lymphocytes and K lymphocytes (also known as T cells and K cells) are another kind of soldier used by the immune system to destroy germs. A product of the lymphatic system, they are transported to the field of battle first by the lymph then by the bloodstream. These T lymphocytes and K lymphocytes attack microbes in close combat. There are other such agents, like the B lymphocytes (or B cells) that act from a distance. B cells produce antibodies, special substances capable of killing the germs responsible for an infection. But these highly effective substances must be carried to the germs, and at the quickest speed possible; microbes have a vexing property of multiplying at great speed and to such proportions that they are beyond the body's ability to produce enough lymphocytes and antibodies to fight them.

Here again, an extremely rapid means of transport is essential, which is achieved by the acceleration of blood flow.

In order to speed the rate of blood circulation, the vessels contract but, more importantly, the heart starts beating at a higher rhythm. While normal cardiac rhythm is 60 beats per minute, during a fever it can elevate to 100 beats per minute or higher. The increased labor of the heart muscles produces heat that contributes to the rise of body temperature. As the bloodstream and everything it transports (red blood cells, platelets, etc.) flows through, rubbing against the vessel walls, more heat is produced. This circulatory escalation is visible on the outside: the individual's skin becomes flushed.

A similar acceleration takes place in the lymphatic system. Normally lymph flows quite slowly through the lymphatic vessels. However, since these vessels are connected to the circulatory system (lymph is continuously flowing into the bloodstream at the level of the subclavian veins) lymph flow speed is dependent upon that of the bloodstream. Now, if the normal lymph output is around 1 quart every twenty-four hours, during a fever it is closer to 2 to 5 quarts that can be discharged into the blood circulation daily. Here, too, the acceleration of movement in the lymph vessels produces heat.

The organs of the body work together, each stepping in at a precise point in the metabolic sequence.

They are each dependent upon one another and must adapt to the activity of their peers. As a consequence, when one of these organs accelerates the speed at which it performs its function, the other organs must do the same. When the heart increases its rhythm, the lungs are forced to increase theirs. Inhalations and exhalations follow each other at a higher rhythm and with greater breadth, which allows for better oxygenation of the blood and faster elimination of carbon dioxide and the wastes it is carrying.

The quantity of undesirable substances the bloodstream transports is greatly increased during a fever. Dead germs are not the only wastes to be eliminated. If an infection was able to develop in the body in the first place, it is because the biological terrain was overrun with metabolic residues and toxins from environmental pollution and the thoughtless ingestion of alcohol, tobacco, drugs, or pharmaceutical medications. All of these harmful substances, which, by creating a favorable environment for germs, have allowed this infection, should also be eliminated. The excretory organs, such as the liver and kidneys responsible for purifying the blood, as well as the sudoriferous and sebaceous glands of the skin, must consequently also escalate their filtering activities to quickly expel wastes from the body. This escalation is yet another source of heat production, which, when added to the others, helps raise the temperature of the body.

The largest wastes in the body must be reduced into smaller particles before they can be expelled by the excretory organs. The "digestion" of these wastes takes place by virtue of a physiological process called *autolysis* in which enzymes break down or destroy them. Countless enzymes throughout the body contribute to this effort, which is also a producer of heat.

In non-infectious fevers—those due to poisoning, overeating, or overwork—the same phenomena take place, although the activity performed by the immune system is a bit more modest. The bulk of the heat engendered will come from autolysis, eliminations, and an overall escalation of metabolic activity.

In summary, we can say that the acceleration of combustions, oxidations, exchanges, transport, purification, eliminations, and so forth that is a natural part of the body's defense process, produces heat, which leads to an elevation in the temperature of the body—in other words, a fever.

To provide a more complete picture, I should also point out that certain germs and white blood cells secrete pyrogenic (fever-inducing) substances. These throw off the body's thermostat, the temperature regulation center located in the hypothalamus. Now adjusted to a temperature higher than the normal 98.6°F to 102°F, for instance—the pace of all metabolic activity escalates to obtain a corresponding body temperature. Generally this irregularity is presented as detrimental, but shouldn't we instead view it as help from nature? By pushing the body to raise its temperature, the microbes are in fact activating the defense system that will bring about their destruction.

THE DIFFERENT KINDS OF FEVER

Because fever is the manifestation of the body's defensive reactions against attack, it does not always appear in the same way. To the contrary, there are numerous different forms fever can take depending on what kind of defensive reactions are implemented by the body.

High or Low-Grade Fevers

Generally speaking, people with strong vitality will experience much more violent and aggressive fevers. They will have a more intense defensive reaction, because they have much more strength at their disposal for guiding it to the best conclusion. A patient lacking vitality, whose body has only a minimal amount of strength for fighting this battle, will produce a weakened defense reaction. Children generally produce higher fevers while the elderly have fevers of much less intensity, because children have more vitality to draw from.

The intensity of the fever also depends on how dangerous the infection is. The more harmful the germs can be to the body and the greater their population, the more likely the body is to react against them in force. If the infection is relatively benign and microbes are not present in large number, the reaction will be reduced proportionately.

Gradual or Sudden Fevers

In gradual fevers, the germs multiply slowly. The microbial invasion is occurring gradually and consequently the problems it causes appear little by little. The fever will take several days to reach its height, and the patient's state follows this evolution. In the beginning he has only slight discomfort brought on by the infection; but this increases from day to day along with the fever.

Abrupt or sudden fevers appear in an entirely different fashion. Here, the multiplication of germs is quite rapid and all the problems and dysfunction caused by the infection appear quickly, suddenly and radically altering the patient's condition. In an hour's time the patient's temperature can shoot up from 98.6°F to 103°F or 104°F. In parallel to this, the state of the infected person can go from normal to the most intense discomfort the disease is capable of producing. This is the case, for example, with yellow fever, an illness that normally rages in certain tropical regions, but it can also be seen in certain kinds of flu.

Fevers That Plateau or Fevers That
Climb Up and Down

Fevers that plateau, with the temperature remaining stable all day, are rather rare. Such a fever would allow us to presume that the microbial threat remained unchanging in its nature, thus the defensive reactions of the body did not differ in their intensity.

Most often, though, the threat posed by germs varies over time. A real battle is taking place between the body and the germs. During these combats, when the winning side begins to tire, the other side can gain the upper hand. Fevers that climb and fall are thus revealing the status of the battle taking place inside the body. If the fever is high, or climbing, it shows that the body is under heavy attack and is strongly fighting back. If the temperature is low, or falling, it means that the germ threat is momentarily vanquished, and the danger it poses is reduced.

Short or Extended Fevers

A fever of short duration shows that the body has quickly neutralized an infection. The defensive mechanisms shut down, because the threat they were responding to has vanished.

When a fever lasts for an extended period, it is a sign that the body has not yet managed to completely defeat the infection, and the defense system must continue its efforts.

Recurring Fevers

Sometimes feverish bouts can recur several times after periods of complete remission. In these cases, although the infection has been properly fought—hence the period of remission—some of the germs responsible for the infection have survived and remain in the depths of the tissue in a dormant state. With the right conditions—such as deterioration of the biological terrain after a period of overwork, intense stress, or a large shock—the germs can emerge from their slumber. Finding themselves in more propitious surroundings, the germs begin to multiply and trigger a new infection.

Intermittent/Relapsing Fevers

These are also bouts of fever that reappear on several occasions but without being separated by a true period of complete remission. The patient has not completely gotten rid of the illness, but her state has temporarily improved between each episode of fever.

These kinds of fever occur when the germ responsible for the infection is difficult for the body to completely destroy and is one that reproduces cyclically. This is the case for the Plasmodium parasite, which is responsible for causing malaria. It colonizes the red blood cells in the bloodstream and multiplies there in vast numbers. After a period of several days, the red blood cells rupture, releasing the parasites back into the bloodstream where they can infect more red blood cells.

The body's defense system is most effective in killing parasites when they are in the blood, not when they are inside the red blood cells. Therefore, the body has strong defensive reactions when the bloodstream is invaded by these parasites and moments of calm when the parasites are inside the red blood cells.

Depending on the specific kind of parasite responsible for causing the malaria, the time necessary for its reproduction and multiplication will be two or three days. The fevers are therefore labeled as *tiertian* or *quartan*, as they will appear on the third or fourth days.

Summary

When the organs are actively working to defend the body against a microbial infection or a poison, an elevation of body temperature will result. If this goes higher than 1.8 degrees above the normal temperature of 98.6°F it is called a fever.

3

The Beneficial Nature of Fever

Fever is generally regarded as an enemy to be fought and defeated. The majority of patients and their families feel fear at the appearance of a fever, a fear that grows stronger with the intensity of the fever and faithfully follows its ups and downs. Fever is far too often identified as the disease itself or its worst aspect, with all therapeutic efforts targeted on getting rid of it. Peace of mind for the patient or the parent of a feverish child returns only when the fever has vanished.

Yet fever is an intentional action produced by the body to defend itself. Fever's beneficial nature has been emphasized by numerous health professionals.

Thomas Sydenham, the seventeenth-century physician known as the father of English medicine, wrote,

"Now, an imposthume [abscess] is the instrument of nature whereby she expels whatever injures the fleshy part, as a fever is her instrument to carry off whatever is prejudicial to the blood. In this case, therefore, it is the business of the physician to assist nature."

According to Paul Carton (1875–1947), one of the great pioneers of natural medicine in France, "Fever simply represents the escalated combustion of bad materials, of poisons put into circulation. It performs a salutary act of neutralizing toxins, a defensive work of metabolic improvement without which wastes could not be accepted and eliminated by the emunctory organs."

Édouard Auber (1804–1873), an expert on the work of Hippocrates, states in his own *Philosophie de la medicine,* "Fever is one of the most powerful healing methods employed by nature."

André Passbecq (1920–2010), one of the best known naturopathic doctors in France, writes "Nothing works as well against illness as a good fever. . . . Fever can be a source of discomfort but, thanks to it, pathogenic substances and toxins are promptly broken down and eliminated. It is a correct action designed to prevent poisoning by cellular toxins, poisons, and infections. The temperature will remain high as long as the bulk of the toxins have not been eliminated."

Naturopath M. Platen wrote, "Fever is an agent of healing and not a specific morbid state of the body." French naturopath Pierre Valentin Marchesseau (1911–

1994) echoes this sentiment: "Fever is a means of self-defense." And American alternative health advocate Herbert M. Shelton (1895–1985) remarked that "fever denotes poisoning."

USING FEVER AS THERAPY

Fever possesses so many therapeutic benefits that a variety of practitioners, aware of its usefulness, have sought means for creating it artificially. These *pyrotherapy* techniques included injections of substances that would not be tolerated by the body in order to force the body to defend itself by creating a fever. The substances used were primarily proteins from milk or other foods, or germs. But why were proteins used?

The human body possesses proteins made from combinations of amino acids specific to each individual. This means that the proteins in the body are different from any proteins it receives from outside. Moreover, the immune system is capable of telling the difference between its own proteins and those of foreign origin.

Of course, foods carry foreign proteins into the body. However, these proteins are normally broken down into amino acids during the digestive process. These amino acids, following their assimilation, are reassembled into proteins specifically designed for the needs of the individual body. Therefore, the food proteins humans receive from external sources only ever enter the blood and tissues in the form of amino acids.

In pyrotherapy the opposite of the natural process is intentionally implemented: proteins are injected directly into the bloodstream. The body feels their presence as a serious threat and unleashes all the means necessary to defend itself: acceleration of blood flow, multiplication of lymphocytes, escalation of metabolic activities, and increased eliminations, all of which, in turn, trigger a fever.

For the most part, these pyrotherapy methods have been abandoned because of the numerous problems they caused due to their anti-physiological nature. The fact remains, nonetheless, that the practice was based on a correct evaluation of the healing virtues of fever.

Fortunately, there is a physiological process that exists for intentionally creating fever: thermal baths, a subject we will revisit in greater depth later. With a hot bath, a person can easily and rapidly escalate and intensify the metabolic activities and defense reactions of the body, which will produce a temporary fever. This method is something that can be turned to for preventive purposes. By correcting the biological terrain, you can prevent illnesses from finding an opportunity to develop.

FEVER IS A WELCOME FRIEND
NOT A FOE TO SLAY

Many people find it surprising that fever can be considered a friend and ally rather than something that should be thwarted. But, as we have seen, fever is evidence of the intense labor performed by the body to break down and eliminate toxic substances and germs. Fever is nothing but the consequence of the defensive activity engendered by the body itself as a means of protection. Countering it would therefore be extremely disadvantageous.

During infectious diseases, the salutary effect of fever is twofold. On the one hand, raising the temperature of the body makes the environment untenable for the germs. These high heats are, in fact, fatal to them. Germs can thrive at the regular body temperature of 98.6°F but let the temperature rise a few degrees to 102°F, 103°F, or 104°F and their living conditions are made adverse to their continued existence. The heat will greatly weaken the germs and severely limit their ability to reproduce.

Fever also alters the living conditions of germs by purifying the terrain, the interior cellular environment of the body. Just like mosquitoes require the stagnant waters of marshes and swamps to thrive, germs need a terrain overloaded with wastes in order to survive and multiply. So, once the biological terrain has been cleansed, it becomes unfavorable for their continued existence and precipitates their disappearance.

Fever is the body's preferred method for treating itself. Consequently, fevers should not be lowered or eliminated thoughtlessly. Cutting a fever short goes against common sense. It would amount to hoping a patient can be cured while opposing every attempt that is made to heal them.

The Benefits of Fever

- Burns away toxins
- Eliminates toxins
- Weakens germs
- Stimulates the immune system
- Accelerates the transportation of lymphocytes to the site of infection

---

Stopping a fever is justified only when the profusion of germs overtaxes the patient's weakened state. If the germs have multiplied in too high a number and are too virulent, the defenses of the patient may no longer be powerful enough to counter them. There is a risk of irreversible and fatal lesions.

In these extreme cases, which are also extremely uncommon, a treatment based on antibiotics and antipyretics is essential. The antipyretic or febrifuge artificially lowers the temperature of the body and provides relief to the patient. Antibiotics will kill the germs in place of the body's defense system. In the majority of cases, though, the fever should be respected; the body is fully capable of stamping out the infection with its own forces. The immune system exists precisely for this purpose.

Halting a fever prevents the body from killing the germs attacking it and from burning away the poisons that are stagnating in its terrain. It also prevents these toxins from being transported to the excretory organs where they can be eliminated. In addition to these toxins that are forced deeper into the tissues, when antipyretics are used the body also has to deal with the poisons imported by these medicines. Abruptly halting the healing process counteracts the body's reactive forces, paralyses its defense system, and breaks the spontaneous forms of resistance it manifests. The toxins produced by the infecting germs and the cadavers of these same germs will not be eliminated properly. The biological terrain remains overloaded, and, consequently, a true healing cannot take place. When the fundamental problem—the deteriorated state of the terrain, which makes it receptive to germs—is not addressed, this will lead to relapses and recurrences, complications and aggravations.

If a flu is cut short, the patient will suffer its lingering effects for the rest of the winter. She will be fatigued and lack vitality because her defense reactions have been smothered. The damaged terrain, which has provided a comfortable bed for the flu, will remain in poor condition. When an upper respiratory tract infection is halted, it will return again and again. If it is again brought to a premature end, bronchitis may result. If this bronchitis is cut short, it may degenerate into pneumonia. The patient will go from one illness to another because the primary disorder, the overloaded biological terrain, remains untreated.

In contrast, what a resurgence of energy, resistance, and joy in living can be experienced when the fever is allowed to do its work.

The propensity to cut fevers short has certainly brought about a diminishing number of acute illnesses, but the consequence of this has been an increase in the number of chronic diseases. By systematically thwarting the body's natural healing efforts, anti-fever therapies that repress symptoms only increase the contaminants in the biological terrain, which, over time, leads to the major lesions and functional disorders of chronic disease.

The objection that is most commonly raised against taking a more respectful approach to fever is based on the danger to the patient's very survival caused by too high a rise in temperature. Of course, this danger is real. But refusing to cut short a fever, in other words, respecting its existence and purpose, does not mean doing nothing. Respecting fever means understanding its action, supporting its work (when, and if, necessary), and temporarily curbing it if it becomes too severe.

Practical means for doing this are provided in the second part of this book.

Summary

Fever is not an enemy to be beaten back; it is simply the consequence of defensive reactions engendered by the body itself. Cutting short a fever means cutting off the work of these natural physical defenses.

4

The Course
of a Fever

In order to support and control a fever, it is necessary
to be able to identify the different stages through which
a fever passes. There are three clearly distinguishable
phases: the period of the fever's onset, the initial rise
(this period is fully established when the fever reaches
its height), and the end phase (which is characterized by
the fall of the body's temperature).

THE ONSET PERIOD

Generally the germs responsible for infections enter the
body in such small number and do not immediately
find favorable conditions for multiplying, so the damage they are able to cause is minimal. It is only when

germs multiply that the damage they cause can become dangerous. The multiplication of germs is a process that can have a protracted duration. A fever can therefore take a few hours or several days to start climbing.

Because the attack made on the body's tissues takes place only gradually, likewise, the work of neutralizing, destroying, and eliminating the germs is implemented little by little. In the beginning, the defense system reactions are neither specific nor localized. The body's defenses are of a general nature at this point, for while the body has detected an infection, the white blood cells have not yet determined the exact nature of the attacker nor the specific measures it needs to implement to fight it.

At this stage of the illness, the symptoms are also of a general nature. The patient has a feeling of general discomfort or overall poor health with aches and restlessness. Sensations of cold, of something irritating the skin, accompanied by shivering may also be present.

THE FEVER'S FULL MANIFESTATION

Once the body's defense systems have been set into motion, their activities gradually escalate. After identifying the attacker, the focus shifts to producing the specific defenses necessary to destroy it. The general intensification of blood circulation, respiration, and the combustion of wastes produces a visible rise in temperature. The fever is now working at full strength. It can spike quickly and then be interrupted by periods of remission, during which time the temperature falls temporarily before climbing back up. This stage can last until the purpose for which the body produced the fever has been achieved.

This purpose is to destroy whatever is threatening the body's physical integrity. The germs need to be killed and their cadavers eliminated, microbial toxins need to be neutralized and expelled, the wastes and residues of the body itself also need to be excreted. When chemical products, venom, or some other poison is responsible for causing the fever, it is these substances that the body must neutralize and eliminate by raising its temperature.

The body must make advance preparations before eliminating all these undesirable substances. They are still too "raw" to be expelled, to borrow Hippocrates' terminology, and therefore still need to undergo the "coction" provided by fever. By "cooking" the wastes in this way, their harmful nature is stripped away and their elimination thus facilitated.

This second phase of fever is therefore characterized by an intense labor to neutralize and break down toxins and poisons before they are truly eliminated from the body.

Because of the toxicity of these poisons, the body retains the maximum amount of water possible in an effort to lessen the concentration of the bodily fluids and reduce the aggressive impact the poisons can have on the tissues and organs. The patient therefore hardly eliminates anything during this time: urinations are rare and he or she barely perspires if at all.

END PHASE

The period at the end of a fever is characterized by strong eliminations and a lowering of the body's temperature. With the toxins neutralized in the preceding stage, the elimination process can at last begin. Evacuation of the dead germs and neutralized poisons is carried out by the excretory organs, the body's normal exit routes. These eliminations can be quite intense as the body violently rids itself of large quantities of poison in a short span of time. Demands are made on all of the organs that eliminate, some more than others depending on the needs of the patient in question.

Abundant perspiration is the most typical form of elimination. The daily volume of sweat excreted can be triple or quadruple the body's normal output, going from 2 or 3 cups a day to 2 or 3 quarts, if not more. The water that had been retained can now leave the body charged with wastes.

These waste-laden fluids also move outward through the urinary glands. There is an increased need to urinate, and the urine produced is copious and dark.

The skin is often the site of cutaneous eruptions affecting the entire surface of the body. The most spectacular example of these eliminations is provided by childhood diseases where, during a bout of measles or chicken pox, for example, children are covered with rashes or pimples. The sudoriferous or sebaceous glands have become congested with the inrush of wastes, causing pimples and red blotches to form.

During this period of exuberant activity by the excretory organs, demands are also made upon the digestive tract. The breakdown and removal of toxins takes place through its mucous membranes. This phenomenon can be observed in the mouth when the tongue becomes glazed with a white coating. The secretions of the salivary glands, the stomach, the liver, and so forth, carry with them not only digestive juices but numerous toxins. This can be detected in the saliva as its taste will change. These wastes are then expelled from the body with the stools. Rapid and copious evacuations of toxins sometimes also take place toward the top of the digestive tract (vomiting) and toward the bottom of the digestive tract (diarrhea).

The respiratory tract also plays a role in this major cleansing process. The breath becomes foul with the gases that are being exhaled. The phlegm formed by the wastes is expectorated, sometimes in impressive quantities.

The Course of a Fever

Onset period: the fever climbs

Full manifestation: the fever hits its peak

End phase: the temperature falls

As toxins and poisons emerge from the depths of the body to be carried to the excretory organs, they necessarily enter into the bloodstream where they drastically alter the composition. It's no longer pure and well-oxygenated blood that is circulating there, it is overloaded with toxic substances. This inevitably has an effect on the patient who can feel all kinds of physical discomfort and mental unease. Her heartbeat becomes erratic and breathing can become difficult; she may feel greatly agitated and anxious.

Fortunately the discomfort experienced during this period will quickly be replaced by a sense of well-being and relaxation when the avalanche of toxins leaving the body has finally passed. When the biological terrain is clean again, the germs infecting it killed and their remains removed, the patient suddenly feels much better. The body's defensive reactions calm down, as evidenced by the fall of the fever's temperature.

In some cases, the intense phase of eliminations truly terminates the illness. The patient needs no more than a few more days of convalescence to recover her full strength. In other cases, one or more additional phases of coction followed by elimination will occur in succession until the terrain has been sufficiently cleansed.

Summary

Fever passes through three stages: In the first it is getting a foothold and establishing itself. In the second the patient experiences spikes in temperature that allow the body to burn off the poisons and germs. The third stage is characterized by strong eliminations of toxins and the fall of the body's temperature back toward its norm.

5

The Dangers
of Fever

Certain symptoms appear when the body can no longer tolerate the intense activity it is housing. It is at this point that fever stops being beneficial and becomes harmful. Allowing the fever to follow its course is no longer a reasonable solution; energetic intervention is called for in order to temper it. (Specific techniques for manipulating fever are explained in part 2, "Controlling Fever.")

Two principal symptoms provide this alert: the fever is either too high or it is lasting for too long a period of time.

AN OVERLY HIGH TEMPERATURE

The ability of each individual's body to handle high temperatures can vary greatly. Some people feel they have reached the end of their rope with a temperature half a degree over 100°F and others not until 104°F. It is therefore difficult to provide a precise figure for "overly high."

Generally speaking, however, we can say that starting at around 102°F the fever is strong and might require intervention to be brought down to a temperature that is less taxing on the patient's resources. The higher the temperature goes beyond this limit, the greater the necessity to moderate it will be.

Any efforts toward lowering a fever should not aim to halt the fever completely but only to reduce its intensity. Totally eliminating a fever amounts to halting all of the body's defensive processes. Fever can be controlled, which is to say it can be allowed to pursue its activities of combustion but at a rate that is more modest than what had been the case; in other words, at a rhythm more compatible with what the patient is capable of tolerating.

Natural medicine has a number of effective methods at its disposal for lowering fever. Because these methods allow the fever to pursue its course, the fever will climb back up again but generally to lesser temperatures than the highs it formerly reached. During the time the fever was more moderate, the patient was able to recover his strength. This momentary respite helps the individual withstand a new intensification of the fever, which is necessary to effectively fight the infection and cleanse the biological terrain.

However high it climbs, the temperature of the new fever spike can also be brought back down to manageable levels again by repeating the techniques initially used. The fever will therefore alternate between periods of intense activity and periods of rest, which permits the patient to allow his fever to continue but at a pace he finds more tolerable.

FEVER WITHOUT REMISSION

Sometimes a fever is not necessarily too high but it lasts for an overly long period of time. Instead of going back down once its peak has been reached and giving way to the copious eliminations that need to take place in the third phase of fever, some fevers are unrelenting and continue burning. The individual will become exhausted and no longer be able to support the effort demanded of the body to complete the cure.

When has a fever gone on for too long? It is difficult to give a hard and fast time limit, as here, too, the tolerance threshold will vary from one individual to the next. Several days will be too long for some people, several hours will tax others beyond their capacity. Furthermore, how high the temperature climbs is a significant factor in what can be tolerated. A person's appearance (clearness of the eyes), the way he feels (clarity of thought), strength levels (exhausted or not), and so forth, are all valuable signals for judging the situation.

While high temperatures are difficult to tolerate, lower grade fevers on a plateau can be equally exhausting. In this latter case, the uncomfortable period lasts longer because the fever does not manage to mature enough to get out of the second stage and trigger the final eliminatory phase.

In this situation, the body is like a smoldering volcano. The coction is taking place but it does not culminate with a liberating explosion, which, in fever, is signaled by copious sweating and eliminations. The entire body is under pressure, toxins are rising from the depths of the tissues, the bloodstream is overloaded with wastes, but they are not expelled from the body. The patient obviously feels terrible and is expending a lot of energy without achieving any result. It is imperative to give assistance to the body at this time so the situation can evolve properly as nature intended. The techniques used in this specific case do not aim at lowering the temperature of the body. To the contrary, more heat (but in moderation) must be supplied to help the fever mature. Additional heat triggers perspiration, which finally gives the overload of toxins a means to exit the body. The other excretory organs will also be triggered to eliminate these poisons.

OTHER SIGNS

There are some additional symptoms that indicate that the patient is overtaxed by fever and swift intervention is called for.

Intense Pain

When the nerve endings in a specific tissue or organ are stimulated too strongly or too intensely, pain will result. This occurs in a number of infections. The numerous microbes and poisons irritate the nerves and tissues, which then become inflamed and painful. One such example would be the painful bronchia of a person suffering from bronchitis.

It is normal for some pain to be felt during an infection. What is not normal is when the pain becomes sharp and persistent. This is a sign that the infectious pocket is attacking the tissues involved too strongly. An additional factor here is the heat of the fever itself, which constitutes another assault on the inflamed tissues, in the same way hot water on a wound is more painful than exposure to lukewarm water.

Spasms

When the body temperature becomes too high, the functioning of the nervous system is upset causing a disruption in the transmission of nerve signals. These distorted signals can cause spasms, in other words, sudden and violent involuntary muscle contractions.

Muscles that are stimulated in this way remain stuck in a contracted state. This situation generally is not long-lasting, but it is still not a pleasant experience. It is a sign that the body is having difficulty tolerating the high temperature of the fever and it is necessary to bring it down.

Delirium

The situation just described concerning the motor nerves is also true for the sensory nerves and the brain. Overheating the neurons of the brain distorts perceptions and disrupts thinking ability. The result is a state of mental confusion, with visual and auditory hallucinations. Thoughts and words may appear to be completely absent of any common sense. Because the patient's motor nerves will also be overstimulated by the high temperature, movements will be disorganized and spasmodic. This unrest should be dealt with quickly by lowering the body temperature.

Fierce Headaches

The headaches that occur during fevers are caused by congestion of the blood vessels that carry the blood through the skull. The heat has a vasodilatory effect. Because they are filled with more blood than normal, the vessels exert an unaccustomed pressure on the surrounding tissues and nerves, which is only aggravated by the fact that these tissues are also themselves dilated by the heat. The pain that results from this congested state can be relieved by applying cold to the body either locally or generally and bringing the patient's temperature down.

Signs That It Is Necessary to Lower a Fever

- When the temperature is too high, starting at about 102°F
- When the fever has no remission
- In the event of intense pain
- In the event of spasms
- In the event of delirium
- In the event of fierce headaches

Summary

By exhausting the patient, fever can become a danger to an individual's health. Fever should be moderated when the temperature rises too high or it drags on for too long a time.

Part Two

Controlling Fever

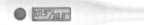

While fever is a powerful healing agent provided by nature, sometimes it acts too strongly for the body to support; on other occasions it labors to fully manifest. It is therefore very important to understand the methods available for moderating fever when necessary as well as those, in the opposing cases, that are capable of stimulating its efforts.

Simple, natural methods exist, which are within everyone's reach. They include measures involving diet, hygiene, hydrotherapy, and techniques for emptying the intestines. The use of medicinal plants with sudorific (sweat-inducing) or febrifuge (fever-reducing) properties as well as those that strengthen the body's defenses can also be added to the mix. All of these different methods can complement each other. Each is important in its own right, of course, and, depending on the patient's specific needs, one will generally be used predominantly.

The illnesses responsible for triggering the healing force of fever can run the full gamut from minor disorders to serious diseases. The recommendations I offer in the following chapters are simply to show what methods are available for controlling fever. While these methods are perfectly applicable for self-use in simple cases, in other, more critical cases, they should not be undertaken by the novice but left to a seasoned health professional.

6

Patient Hygiene

Properly speaking, hygiene is not a therapy, but by contributing to the patient's well-being, it has a healing effect all the same. Measures as simple as good physical hygiene (rest, airing out the room, and so forth) and good mental hygiene (stress reduction, elimination of noises, establishing inner calm) spare the strength of the patient and thereby support the task on which the body is working: healing. Rather than fighting against problems that can cause fatigue, such as dealing with the cold, the body can devote all its energy to fighting against the illness. The body's forces will be concentrated rather than scattered dealing with a variety of issues.

So what are some of these hygiene measures we can utilize?

REST

During a fever, great demands are made on the patient's forces. A great deal of energy is expended to permit the healthy escalation of metabolic activity as well as that of the immune system's defenses. It is therefore greatly preferable that the patient rest rather than pursuing his usual activities. By doing this, his energies will all be concentrated on a single goal.

Rest—rest in bed—is therefore compulsory. The patient should be comfortably settled in a horizontal position. There should be plenty of covers so that he can add more if he feels a chill, something that is quite common during the onset of illness.

The room temperature should be pleasant. It should not be too cold, which will force the body to expend needless energy trying to stay warm; nor should it be too hot, which will exhaust the patient for no good purpose.

Recommendations for getting plenty of rest are not restricted to just the body; the mind, too, needs to take it easy. The room should be peaceful, which means sheltered as much as possible from the hubbub of daily life and noise. Distractions such as radio, television, and electronic games should be avoided, as they will subtract from the patient's strength without offering anything positive in return with respect to healing. Inner tranquillity, or at least a little peace of mind, will promote and encourage the unrestricted performance of the body's organic processes. The people around the patient can contribute to this state by remaining calm and confident themselves.

AIR CIRCULATION

The room in which the patient is resting should be aired out on a regular basis. The patient needs oxygen and, therefore, clean, pure air. The body is working at an elevated rhythm and expelling large amounts of gaseous waste that are harmful to the body. The bad breath of those suffering from illness is evidence of this intense elimination of poisons. When it evaporates, the perspiration covering the patient's skin also spreads waste products in a volatile form throughout the room. In combination with those released from the lungs, they contribute to creating the strong, disagreeable odor that characterizes the poorly aired rooms of sick people.

When the room is being ventilated, which should occur every few hours, precautions should be taken to ensure that the patient doesn't become cold.

HYDRATION

A patient burning with fever can easily do without food, but she must drink. The ideal beverage for those suffering from fever is water.

Patients will need to replace the fluids they are losing through perspiration and urination. Sufficient fluid in the tissues is essential for cellular exchanges to take place properly and for the metabolism to function correctly. A dehydrated body functions in slow motion and is ill equipped to defend itself.

Regular water intake also reduces the concentration of toxins in the bloodstream and the cellular fluids, lessening their ability to damage the tissues. Abundant intake of liquids also makes it possible for the body to transport the wastes to the excretory organs where they can be evacuated from the body. If the quantities of sweat and urine are reduced because of a lack of liquid, the amount of waste the body eliminates will also be reduced.

A continuous transit of liquid has both a vitalizing and cleansing effect and is necessary for the body to mount the best defense against an illness. The beverages used for this purpose should be non-nutritious, because the body's digestive abilities are weakened during a fever. They should not provide an additional intake of toxins either, as is the case with coffee, black tea, and commercial sodas.

The beverages that are recommended during the course of a fever are therefore:

Water. This can be either tap water or bottled spring water. It should be drunk cold or at room temperature, depending on the patient's prefer-ence. The patient should trust her instincts and drink as much as she wants. If the individual is drinking too little, she should be encouraged to drink; regularly offer her a glass of water over the course of the day.

Herbal Teas. Although they contain a variety of sub-stances from the medicinal plants they are brewed from, herbal teas generally lack any nutrients (as long as they are not sweetened with sugar). They have a pleasant aroma and taste that, depending on the case, can have a soothing or stimulating effect. The most highly recommended herbal teas to drink during a fever are those with linden, mint, verbena, and chamomile.

CLEANLINESS

A feverish patient can release several quarts of sweat a day (in comparison to the 2 or 3 cups worth that a healthy person generally excretes). This perspiration is also more charged with wastes than ordinarily because of the body's efforts to detoxify itself. These wastes will quickly soak into the pajamas and bed sheets.

To avoid having the patient lying in the wastes that have been expelled through the skin and, more impor-tantly, to avoid reabsorption of these toxins by pro-longed contact, it is essential that the patient regularly wash herself and change what she has been wearing. The sheets on the patient's bed should be replaced by clean ones as often as necessary. This will increase the patient's comfort and also prevent reabsorption of the wastes that were most recently expelled.

Here, too, precautions should be taken to avoid the patient becoming too cold while the bed is being remade or while she is changing her clothes.

MOVEMENT

The desire to be moving or to be doing something does not generally appear during the first two phases of fever. During the fever's onset and the time when it spikes to its highest temperature, the patient feels sapped by the illness and usually just wants to remain lying down above all else. The desire to get moving reappears most often during the third stage, the time when the body's temperature is returning to normal.

While remaining in bed and resting during the course of a short fever (such as the flu, which usually lasts three to four days) is beneficial because it allows the patient to save his strength, this is not true for fevers that last longer. The spikes and drops in temperature that are characteristic of the second and third stages of a fever can occur repeatedly for a week or more. Remaining confined to bed for a period that long can have adverse consequences.

The body's metabolic activities slow down during a prolonged absence of any physical activity. Breathing, circulation, and cellular exchanges will occur at a slower rate and with less intensity. This, in turn, creates a sense of fatigue that engenders a loss of enthusiasm and tone. To fight the forces of inertia and keep the gears of the body's engine in good working order, modest physical activity may be called for.

Movement has a stimulating effect on all the body's organic functions. The heart beats with greater intensity, which activates the blood circulation, which, in turn, permits irrigation of the depths of the body's tissues. The lungs breathe more deeply creating better oxygenation. Exchanges are encouraged and toxins are more effectively broken down and eliminated. In short, we could say that external movement (muscle contraction) stimulates internal movement (metabolic activities).

Consequently, a little movement is sometimes necessary over the course of an illness before healing is complete. Taking a few steps back and forth in the bedroom or walking up and down the hall will allow the patient to activate his metabolism. This brings the body out of the state of stagnation and lethargy that occurs by remaining immobile for too long and triggers renewed activity in organ function and the body's immune system.

The patient should move around just long enough to

get the body stimulated but no more. Extending activity beyond this point will simply be exhausting.

INTESTINAL CLEANSING

Encouraging intestinal cleansing is only necessary for those patients suffering from constipation. Intestines that have not been emptied for two or three days will be filled with wastes. As we have seen, during a fever the body's efforts are aimed at burning off and eliminating anything that is foreign to it, in other words, the wastes, wherever they may be located in the body. The wastes imprisoned in the intestines will not be exempt. These stagnant intestinal wastes are even more harmful to the body at this time, because the fever will raise the temperature of the intestines, which only encourages the fermentation and putrefaction of the fecal matter thereby increasing the quantity of poisons in the body.

The intestinal poisons must be neutralized and eliminated, which requires intensive labor on the body's part as the intestines can easily contain from 2 to 4 pounds of material. Burning away these wastes also requires an intensification of metabolic activity, which has repercussions on body temperature. As long as these wastes remain in the body, the fever will be pushed higher (or at least remain at its upper levels).

In this situation, the simplest means of providing

relief to the body consists of intentionally emptying the intestines. The strength that will be saved by doing this can then be made available for destroying germs and cleansing the biological terrain. The immune system can concentrate all its forces on microbes rather than on wastes that are easy to eliminate.

The laxatives used to empty the intestines should be mild. A strong laxative will cause too much irritation to the intestines. The body will then react forcefully to the additional attack, causing the fever to climb higher.

A laxative can be mild and still be quite effective. Those whose action is most easy to tolerate include:

Castor Oil. While most laxatives work by stimulating the peristaltic activity of the end of the colon, castor oil works on the small intestine. In the past castor oil was taken by the spoonful and swallowed straight. Because of its extremely unpleasant taste, it has created bad memories for generations of children. The obstacle posed by its foul taste is no longer any hindrance since it is now available in capsules. One dose should be all that is required, but the dosage depends on the size of the capsules. Follow the manufacturer's instructions.

Alder Buckthorn. The bark of this common tree has laxative properties that are so gentle it can even be tolerated by pregnant women. Using a mother tincture rather than tablets or pills makes it easier to tailor the dosage more precisely for the individual's needs. Take 40 to 70 drops of the mother tincture mixed with water. It will take several hours to take effect.

Golden Shower Tree (*Cassia fistula*). This is a mild laxative that is pleasant to take. The plant produces a fruit (which can be found inside the pod); three slices of this sweet fruit should be sufficient to stimulate the intestines. This plant can also be prepared as a tea or decoction; add 1¾ ounces of crushed pods to a pint of water and boil for ten minutes.

Mallow. Mallow is a gentle, nonirritating laxative that is recommended for cases of chronic constipation (atonic or spasmodic), especially when the digestive tract is inflamed. It can be taken as an infusion: 1 ounce of flowers or leaves should be added to 1 quart of water and left to steep for ten to twelve minutes. This will provide 1 or 2 cups of tea. Mallow is also available in tablet form: dosage is generally 2 or 3 tablets; follow manufacturer's instructions. If using a mother tincture, put 20 to 50 drops in a glass of water.

These are only a few suggestions out of many options. If the patient customarily uses another plant or preparation and knows what the proper dose is for a gentle but effective laxative action, by all means con-

tinue using that preparation. Because it is already famil-
iar to the patient, she will find it easier to work with.

Summary

Good patient hygiene involving rest, calm, a well-aired
room, and so forth contributes greatly to the patient's
well-being and thereby to his cure.

7

Controlling Fever with Hydrotherapy

The regulation of body temperature takes place primarily through the skin, which is also the organ that is chiefly involved in hydrotherapeutic applications.

When the body has collected too much heat, as is the case with any strenuous physical effort, but also with fevers, it is the skin that, by opening up and perspiring, permits the loss of the excess heat. Conversely, when the body is cold, it is again the skin with its large absorbent surface, that makes it possible for heat (such as from a hot bath) to enter the body.

The skin's great capacity for absorption comes from the fact that it has such a rich vascular network, an extremely developed grid of capillaries that irrigates the entire body surface. Capillaries are extremely thin blood vessels. They are often compared to hairs (hence their name, from the Latin word for hair, *capillaris*); yet in reality they are much thinner than hairs. Although they are small in size, they are great in number. They also possess the ability to dilate enormously: their dimensions can double and even triple in size! A considerable amount of the volume of blood circulating through the entire body can be found in the skin. It has been calculated that, when circumstances call for it, a full 20 percent of the body's blood will be drawn into the skin—an enormous amount. The bloodstream is the greatest conductor of heat in the body. When heat touches the skin, the blood will absorb that warmth and transport it to the rest of the body. Similarly, when the skin makes contact with a source of cold, the blood will transport heat to the affected areas, thus causing the body to lose heat overall.

Hydrotherapy methods are among the best means we have for controlling heat flow. But why should we resort to water, wouldn't the use of warm air be just as effective and simpler?

It is possible for the body to absorb and lose heat through air's contact with the skin. However, this contact is less intense than when the temperature source is a denser material (like water). In fact, the denser the material, the greater the temperature transfer. The skin can tolerate contact with air that is above 176°F, as in a sauna, because the temperature transfer is weak. Your skin would never be able to stand contact with water of that temperature. It would have even less tolerance of a solid object that had been heated that hot, such as a piece of metal. When it comes to cold temperatures, contact with an ice cube chills the skin more than contact with ice-cold water, which, in turn, provides a greater transfer than contact with air of the same temperature. Using water therefore combines great effectiveness with easy handling.

At first glance, hydrotherapy methods can appear to lack exactitude. In reality, they can be adjusted infinitely depending on how warm or cold the water is, the extent of skin surface covered or not by the water, and the length of time the patient spends in the water.

The hydrotherapy methods presented in this chapter use cold water to lower the body temperature when a fever climbs too high and use hot water to help the fever do its work. These methods are by no means the only ones. There are many different methods as well as ways to apply them. I have chosen the simplest techniques here so that patients and caregivers can quickly put them to use.

REDUCING FEVER

When cold water is applied to the skin, the body loses heat and becomes colder. This cooling effect is physiological (in accord with normal body functioning) up to a certain limit. Beyond this limit, the cold paralyzes the cells, slowing their rate of functioning. If contact with the source of cold is prolonged, the cells located even deeper in the body will also cool down and their activity will diminish. The body will be forced to take action to protect itself. It does this, in part, by exporting warm blood from deeper in the body to the portion of skin exposed to the cold. This defensive reaction will continue for as long as the contact with the cold water continues.

This is how, by artificially "endangering" the skin with the hydrotherapeutic application of cold water, the body can be induced to give up some of its heat in a continuous manner. I will provide four different procedures here for reducing the temperature of a fever, beginning with the gentlest and ending with the most energetic application.

Cold Rub

A cold rub is the gentlest procedure and consequently the one that subtracts the least amount of heat from the body. The technique consists of cupping your hand and filling it with a small amount of cold water, which is then spread over the skin. Rubbing in a way that does not apply too much friction, you make sure the water is evenly distributed. Normally the rub is done with bare hands. When used on a bedridden patient, it is better to apply the water with a small washcloth or sponge.

If using a washcloth, dip it in cold water (between 59°F and 68°F*) and wring it out very lightly. Begin by rubbing one arm, starting at the hand and working up to the shoulder. Do the same on the other arm before applying water to the legs, one at a time, working from the foot up to the hip. Next, lightly rub the patient's back, and then finish the session by working on the front of the torso.

When the patient's health is fragile and he exhibits a lack of vitality, the part of the body being worked on should be uncovered and then covered back up before proceeding to the next area. This will prevent the patient from getting too cold, which could diminish the effectiveness of the treatment. With more robust patients, keeping covered is not necessary; exposure to the ambient cool air will actually enhance the cooling effect of this treatment.

The cold rub should take only a few minutes. The patient should then get back under the covers. A large amount of water is not called for here. The skin should be just slightly moistened with the cold water. Because of how it is evenly spread on the skin with the light friction of the rubbing, the water will disperse in a thin film that the body's heat will have no trouble evaporating in a short while. Even though this treatment is brief, the application of cold water to the

*Using a food thermometer can be a convenient way to measure the water temperature if your normal thermometer doesn't measure these cooler temperatures.

skin will remove some heat from the body and lower the temperature of the fever. This method can be used several times a day, depending on the needs and condition of the patient.

Wrapping the Calves

This application consists of enveloping each calf with a large washcloth or hand towel that has been soaked in cold water (between 59°F and 68°F) and gently wrung out.

The patient should be lying stretched out on a bed with a folded bath towel placed beneath her calves to prevent water from dripping onto the bedding. The first calf should be wrapped in the cold cloth, covering the area from the ankle to the base of the knee. Next do the same to the second calf before covering both with a dry towel and pulling the covers back over the patient.

Although the calves represent only a small portion of the body's surface, they have a large quantity of blood vessels so a substantial amount of heat can be released this way. The effect of this treatment is obviously more restrained than it would be if a larger portion of the body was in contact with these cold cloths. Furthermore, the patient will not need to get out of bed or uncover too much of herself. More benefit will be provided by this treatment if, after several minutes (anywhere from three to ten), the wrapping is changed; by this point the initial wrapping will have collected too much heat to provide any cooling effect.

Depending on both how high the patient's temperature is and the strength of her forces, this technique can be repeated two or three times successively. Despite its simplicity, this procedure is amazingly effective when it comes to bringing down dangerously high fevers. It is especially recommended for treating children.

To amplify the effects of this treatment, vinegar can be added to the water that is being used (2 parts water to 1 part vinegar). In Europe this treatment is called "vinegar booties." The slightly irritating effect of the vinegar on the skin prompts an additional flow of blood to the surface, which increases the amount of blood that is brought into contact with the cold.

The Torso Bathing Suit

This treatment is a bit more "athletic" for the patient: it works on the torso, where the majority of the internal organs are housed. The torso is also the part of the body where the most heat is stored.

A bath towel should be spread over the bed to protect it from dripping water. Next a second bath towel, one that is large enough to wrap around the patient's torso one and a half times, should be dipped in cold water (59°F to 68°F) and then lightly wrung out. With the patient sitting up in bed, wrap his torso with the wet towel. The towel should extend from beneath the armpits to the hips. Next take the dry towel that was spread over the bed and wrap it around the wet towel. Then have the patient lie back down in the bed under one or two covers. The more water contained in this "torso bathing suit," and the colder it is, the more heat it will remove from the body. But, here, as elsewhere, take care not to overdo things.

Using the coldest water possible and then not wringing enough out of the towel can have harmful effects. The patient's strength should always be figured into the equation. There's a difference between causing a chill to bring a fever down, and making the patient cold. Too much cold applied to the body for too long a time will not only remove the excess heat of the fever but steal the body's normal heat as well. As happens whenever someone gets too cold, the body loses strength, the metabolism is disrupted, and the defense system's powers are reduced—all things that need to be absolutely avoided during a fever.

It will take anywhere from three to ten minutes for the torso wrapping to become warm. It will have a soothing effect on the patient at this point, so it should not be removed in one fell swoop. However, it must be removed before it becomes cold again and makes the patient cold, which is what will happen if it's left on for more than twenty minutes to an hour.

A substantial amount of heat can be removed from the body thanks to this torso bathing suit method. However, it may be necessary, with high fevers, for example, to perform this treatment two or three times a day.

The Lukewarm Demi-bath

In this treatment, the patient sits in a bathtub that has been filled with just enough water to reach the bottom of the rib cage. This means that only the bottom half of the body is in direct contact with the water. The temperature of the water should be around 77°F; for weaker patients, the temperature can be up to 95°F. The bath should last from one to five minutes, again depending on the patient's vitality, and may be done once or twice a day. Do not extend this time frame; it can weaken the patient.

A variation of this treatment consists of starting the bath at 95°F and then making it gradually cooler by adding cold water.

ENCOURAGING FEVER

While, because of its many blood vessels, the skin is capable of ridding the body of excess heat, for the same reason it is also capable of absorbing large amounts of heat.

When placed in contact with heat, the temperature of the peripheral layers of the skin will rise. The constantly circulating bloodstream will then take this heat and transport it inside the body. When this levy of heat is continued for a sufficient amount of time, the body's temperature will rise proportionately, which naturally supports and accelerates metabolic activities.

This simple means for amplifying the body's working rhythm is quite a useful tool to be aware of. In some patients, while the body is certainly defending itself, it is at a rhythm that is too weak and too slow. The fever doesn't develop and the saving spike of fever, which is saving because of the period of intense eliminations that follows it, does not happen. The patient remains stuck in the first stage of the fever and cannot progress to the second and third phases.

This generally occurs when the patient lacks strength. Fortunately this deficiency can be easily addressed by donating energy to the patient in the form of heat. This heat will intensify metabolic activity and strengthen the work of the immune system; in other words, the fever will now perform its work properly.

One gentle manner of providing heat to the patient is a total dry wrap.

Total Dry Wrap

To encourage fever with this method, spread two wool blankets over the bed and lay a sheet on top of them. The patient should lie down, naked, on top of the sheet with arms extended overhead. Grasp the left side of the sheet and wrap it around the patient's chest and left arm. Have the patient lower her arms and extend them along her torso. The upper end of the sheet should then be wrapped around the chest, above both arms; wrap the lower end around the right leg. This wrapping should be quite tight at the throat and feet to prevent any cold air from getting in. Place two hot water bottles next to the patient, one on either side of the torso. Then fold the two wool blankets over the patient's body.

Heat will be provided to the patient not only by the hot water bottles but by her body as well. Heat that is normally lost through the skin is retained by the sheet and blankets. As the patient's body temperature gradually rises, so will the body's defense system activities. Allow for a strong period of perspiration before stopping the treatment. Three quarters of an hour to two hours is generally a sufficient period of time.

Summary

Cold hydrotherapy applications make it possible to control a fever, which means lowering it without killing it, when it is too high. Application of heat provides a means of encouraging fevers that aren't developing.

8

Diet and Fever

The way a patient is nourished during a fever is a complete therapy in its own right if used properly. A restrictive diet, or even fasting, and the reintroduction of food at an opportune moment can both be a large help in bringing down a fever. But how does this work?

WHEN TO FAST AND WHEN TO EAT

Following the initial onset of fever, the patient generally does not feel hungry and will willingly go without food. But just because he is not receiving any energy does not mean the body is not expending it. Because of the acceleration of all metabolic activities, the body is actually working at a stronger rhythm and expending quite a bit of energy.

In the beginning, the body makes use of the nutritive

87

substances that the patient consumed in the days before the fever. The body also draws from glycogen reserves stored in the liver and muscles. It can also take advantage of nutrients that result from the breakdown of wastes, which releases amino acids, minerals, and a number of other substances the body can recycle.

While these means are sufficient at the beginning of a fever to maintain the body's energy levels, this will no longer be the case after several days. The body soon reaches the end of its reserves and finds itself threatened by malnutrition. The speed at which this point is reached depends on the individual. Undernourishment deprives the body of the nutrients it needs to cover its basic energy needs as well as what is needed to repair tissues and defend against the infection. To avoid entering a malnourished state, the body must resort to an emergency measure to get the nutrients it requires: *autolysis*.

Autolysis is a process in which the organism digests (*lysis*) its own tissues (*auto*). Enzymes break down the proteins in the tissues into amino acids, fatty acids, glucose, and so forth. But the autolysis process does not just casually attack any tissue. The least essential are targeted before the more important ones. In this way, thanks to the natural intelligence that governs all body processes, autolysis first breaks down the wastes and poisons lying stagnant in the biological terrain and then the diseased tissues before it will turn to the tissues that make up the essential organs of the body.

Autolysis is an active process, and, as such, it requires an expenditure of energy. Occurring during a fever and aiming to avoid a dangerous situation (malnutrition), it takes place with a certain amount of intensity. There's an acceleration of metabolic activities, which increases the body's temperature, which, in turn, will cause the fever to climb. The intensity of this temperature rise will be facilitated by the immune system, which is also working hard to combat the multiplication of germs brought about by undernourishment and deficiencies. As we have already seen, the more the body's forces shrink the greater those of the germs increase.

A patient may therefore go from a fever caused by overload (of wastes, poisons, germs) to one caused by deficiency (of nutrients) without any clearly perceivable transition. Because the causes of these two fevers are different, the means to control them will also be different. While a restrictive diet was helpful for a while, all at once a reintroduction of food will be needed so that the body can avoid malnutrition.

The reintroduction of a carefully chosen food will reduce the fever caused by autolysis. But taking this step prematurely, when the fever is still in the phase caused by overload, will not have a positive effect whatsoever. When the body's main concern is burning excess wastes, the digestive tract will be in no condition to digest properly. Giving the patient something to eat at this juncture, in a misguided effort to ensure he keeps his strength, will actually cause his condition to deteriorate. The poorly digested or undigested foods will only create new wastes for the body to neutralize and eliminate. As the body must increase its efforts, the temperature rises.

Giving the patient something to eat at the wrong time is equivalent to throwing oil on a fire. Good diet management is therefore a complete means in its own right to controlling fever. But what foods are appropriate?

DIET DURING A FEVER:
THE THREE STAGES

While it is normal for someone at the beginning of a fever to be satisfied with only drinking fluids, this state cannot last long. After a period of time—which will vary from one person to the next—the body's reserves will become depleted and some food intake will be essential. However, because of the period of not eating that characterizes the beginning stage of a fever, the digestive tract will have been left idle and will need to be brought back to normal functioning gradually.

The recommended diet for someone with a fever includes three distinct stages:

1. Liquid stage
2. Fluid stage
3. Solid stage

The diet begins with the simplest and least nutritious, progressing from the easiest to digest to the most nutritious. Following the absence of any food except for drinks (liquid stage), foods should be reintroduced in an extremely diluted form (fluid stage). This helps the digestive tract emerge from its torpor and gradually become capable of digesting foods with greater consistency (solid stage).

We'll now take a closer look at each of these stages—what each consists of, its purpose, and how to tell when it should make way for the following stage.

The Liquid Stage

The liquid stage consists of ingesting drinks exclusively. The purpose of this is to provide the body the liquid it needs to function properly while avoiding any nutritive intake.

For this reason, drinks containing protein are excluded. It used to be common practice to give patients beef or vegetable bouillon mixed with a beaten egg to fortify them during a fever. Proteins encourage the assimilation of other nutrients. Fats, minerals, and carbohydrates are integrated into the tissues more thoroughly when proteins are present. In fact, proteins form a framework in the tissue that nutrients can adhere to, much the same way that fish are caught in the mesh of a net. This fixative role played by proteins runs directly counter to the body's objective for triggering a fever, which is to extract toxins and poisons out of the tissue so they can be expelled.

In addition to protein drinks, all beverages that contain too many nutriments, in other words, those containing sugars (sweetened herbal tea, juice, soda) or fats (milk), or those containing toxins (coffee, black tea, alcohol), are contraindicated because they place too high a demand on the digestive capabilities of the patient; and, in the case of the latter beverages, their intoxicating effect is not at all helpful.

The beverages that *are* recommended are as follows.

Tap or Spring Water. Water should be the principal drink. It is good to drink from 2 to 3 quarts a day to make up for the liquid lost in sweat.

For those who also wish to drink something with a little flavor, homemade vegetable broths and herbal teas are good additions.

Herbal Tea. Chamomile, verbena, lime blossom, mint, or any other unsweetened herbal tea is acceptable.

Vegetable Broth. The broth should be light and should contain no flour or grains. Place 2 pounds of potatoes, 1 pound of carrots, several lettuce leaves, and ¼ pound leeks in enough water (about 1½ quarts) so that after one hour of cooking, the volume is about a quart or a little more. Strain the solid parts from the broth before drinking it.

Salt should only be added for those individuals with low blood pressure.

Rice Water. When a fever is accompanied by severe diarrhea, it is a good idea to reduce it (but not eliminate it entirely) with the help of rice water. Rice water can be prepared by boiling 2½ tablespoons of rice in 1 quart of water for half an hour and then straining and drinking the liquid.

The liquid stage guidelines can be altered slightly for children, who should not be denied nutritive intake at this stage in their lives.

Milk. For children who are accustomed to drinking it regularly, milk, preferably diluted with water, is acceptable.

Vegetable and Fruit Juices. Juices are the most nutritious beverages. They are recommended for children, who, generally speaking, cannot tolerate a restrictive diet, and for adults who cannot get by on only water but who are not yet ready to move on to the fluid stage. These juices should be 100 percent juice with no sugar added and should be drunk slightly diluted with water. Fruit and tomato juices should be reserved for those people who have no problem metabolizing fruit acids.* If making your own juice, be sure that the fruits from which the juices are made are ripe.

---

*See Christopher Vasey, *The Acid-Alkaline Diet for Optimum Health: Restore Your Health by Creating pH Balance in Your Diet* (Rochester, Vt.: Healing Arts Press, 2nd edition, 2006).

How long should the liquid stage last? Given the fact that digestive capabilities are reduced when body temperature is rising, the liquid stage should be adhered to until the temperature begins to come down again, at which point the fluid stage should be adopted. In practice, the liquid stage can also be interrupted if the patient is getting weak from hunger. The main criterion to apply here is the patient's condition. As long as the patient is doing well on the liquid diet and is not pained by hunger, it should be followed without any changes.

For people whose biological terrain has been greatly compromised by toxin overload (from overeating) and/or poison overload (from tobacco, alcohol, etc.), the liquid diet provides a marvelous opportunity for cleansing while also supporting the body's own efforts to detoxify using fever.

For young children, the liquid stage should last between twelve and thirty-six hours—no longer. Because their bodies' reserves are necessarily much smaller, children need to receive more substantial foods much sooner than adults to avoid malnutrition.

In determining when to move to the next stage, the desire to ingest something more nutritious is also an important sign that should be taken into consideration. However, this desire must be satisfied gradually. Going directly from the liquid diet to solid foods will overtax the body's digestive capabilities. The fluid stage is an important step.

The Fluid Stage

In the fluid stage, the foods ingested have more consistency than in the liquid stage, but they are not yet solid foods.

The drinks ingested in the previous stage (water, broth, etc.) can be thickened with grains or a flour-based product. This means the addition of starch, a slow sugar, but still precludes the addition of protein and fatty foods. The preparation should be only lightly salted. The starch food that is easiest on the digestive tract is tapioca. But you can also use potatoes, wheat flour, semolina, cream of rice, and small pastas such as vermicelli. Only a small amount of this starch ingredient should be used. In the beginning, for example, use no more than 1 or 2 teaspoons for a bowl of soup. The amounts can be gradually increased but care should be taken to make sure the preparation remains mostly fluid.

There are two other options that are acceptable at this stage: crushing a ripe banana and leaving it in the open air for fifteen minutes before eating so that it becomes quite sweet and selecting a completely ripe (to avoid ingestion of acids) apple and eating it freshly grated.

When the fluid diet has been introduced at the right time, it will be evident by the patient's renewed strength and by an improvement in her overall condition. If the time is not right, the fever will start climbing again and the patient's overall condition will worsen. This indicates that the liquid diet was abandoned too soon and should be resumed.

How long should the fluid stage last? Here, too, this depends on the patient: she should remain on the fluid diet for as long as it feels good. Hunger, any weakness caused by a lack of food, and a desire for something more nutritious are signs that the time has come to move on to the solid food stage.

The Solid Food Stage

The first two stages were characterized in part by an absence of any protein intake, which, as previously explained, makes it easier for the body to separate and remove the wastes and poisons burdening the internal cellular environment. While this was beneficial while the fever was high and actively burning off toxins, this is no longer the case after the fever has passed. The patient has been weakened by his battle and now needs fortification through the intake of solid food.

In this stage protein intake is not only beneficial (because it restocks the body's reserves and renews the patient's strength) it is essential for encouraging the tissues to utilize the fats, minerals, and vitamins entering the body.

To provide the convalescent patient proper nourishment, meals must be well-balanced, containing protein foods as well as starchy foods and other low-fat foods. For example, a piece of cheese or an egg can serve as the protein food, potatoes or pasta can serve as a starch, and vegetables can accompany the meal as a source of minerals. In the beginning the meals should be light and simple, only gradually becoming heavier and more nutritional.

The lightest proteins, in other words, the first to be introduced back into the diet, should be cheeses—starting with softer cheeses such as goat's or farmer's cheese and progressing to harder cheeses such as Swiss. Eggs shouldn't be introduced right away and should first be incorporated in fluid form, such as in a soup, before being eaten straight with other foods. Meat and fish should only be introduced afterward, once the patient is ready to resume his normal diet, except in the case of heavy meat eaters whose bodies, because of deficiency problems, might need their proteins more quickly.

How long should the solid food stage of the treatment be followed? While this question may appear surprising, it needs to be addressed. It may happen that the introduction of solid food occurred prematurely. If the patient's temperature rises during this period and some of his other symptoms reappear, you must reverse the treatment and return to a fluid diet, which will be more suitable for the patient's actual condition.

Mistakes like this are always possible when caring for someone suffering from fever. The moment to actually make the step from one dietary stage to the next is sometimes difficult to determine. The adverse or beneficial reactions are not always foreseeable; trial and error will always be the best way to proceed.

Naturally, if the transition to solid food leads to a general state of feeling better, it should be continued in this direction, albeit gradually, until the individual can fully resume his normal diet.

Foods can, and should, be used therapeutically to soothe fever and reduce the intensity of a patient's symptoms. The way people suffering from fever are fed—gradually taking them from liquids to thicker fluids like pureed broths and then solid foods, with the option of going in the other direction if a stage of the treatment was introduced too soon—is something that can contribute greatly to healing. This commonsense way of proceeding forms a middle ground between two overly extreme paths: the total fast, which can easily lead to malnutrition, or a diet of solid foods, which at the height of a fever will only increase its intensity.

Summary

The recommended diet during a fever consists of three stages: a liquid stage, fluid stage, and solid food stage.

9

Intestinal Drainage

Sometimes, some of the temperature spikes occurring during a fever are not due to germs but are caused by the toxic wastes that are poisoning the body. Among these, intestinal wastes figure prominently.

The intestines consist of a tube about 18 feet long (the small intestine) and one that is 5 feet in length (the colon, or large intestine). The diameter of the intestines can vary between 1 and 3 inches. A large and varied quantity of matter can lie stagnant in the intestines. When daily eliminations do not occur, fermentation and putrefaction can easily result because of the heat and humidity that governs this region of the body. A large number of toxins can be produced this way, increasing the level of the body's poisoned state. The efforts the body makes in its attempt to neutralize and eliminate these wastes will be added to those it is making to kill the germs. All this can lead to a rise in temperature.

In this situation, emptying the intestines with the aid of one of the enema methods described in this chapter will provide rapid relief to the body and a lowering of the fever. An enema consists of introducing water into the intestines so that the stools are liquefied, which facilitates their evacuation. The two methods described here, the rectal douche and the 1-quart enema are particularly easy and provide quick results. Both methods can be performed by the patient in privacy; no assistance is needed.

THE RECTAL DOUCHE

The rectal douche is the mildest type of enema. The amount of water injected into the anus fills only the bottom end of the colon: the rectal ampulla. The water is introduced with the help of a bulb-style enema syringe that contains a little over 1 cup of water (3 deciliters, to be precise).

The rectal douche allows rapid, easy introduction of water into the colon, water which, when expelled, creates a vacuum and draws down the fecal matter located higher in the intestines. The abrupt evacuation of the water and fecal matter that results triggers intestinal peristalsis, pushing the other matter out of the body.

Care should be taken to make sure the syringe is completely full of water in order to avoid the injection of any air. The water used should be at body temperature.

Perform this operation as follows: Inject the water into the anus with the enema syringe while standing up. Once the water has been injected, remove the cannula and sit down on the toilet. Do not try to hold the water in; it should come out all at once. The douche should be performed two or three times in a row. The water expelled will be clearer each time, showing that the colon has been partially cleansed of the wastes burdening it.

THE 1-QUART ENEMA

This enema fills the descending colon with water. The water that is introduced can flow by its own weight once you are seated on the toilet, which is not the case with enemas that use several quarts of water.

The materials necessary for this enema can be found in a complete enema kit, which can be purchased at a drugstore or any medical supply store. It includes a container for the water, a long rubber tube, and a cannula equipped with a faucet. Fill the container with water that has been warmed to body temperature and place it on a table or dresser. Thanks to the force provided by its own weight, the water will easily make its way into the intestines. The cannula should be placed in the anus

with the faucet closed. Open the faucet only after getting down on all fours and leaning your head and torso
forward to facilitate the water's penetration.

Sometimes, to further facilitate this penetration, it
may be necessary to change position to some degree or
take deep breaths. If the water pressure becomes too
strong or painful, the flow of liquid can be halted by
closing the faucet.

Once all the water has been introduced into the
colon, the cannula should be withdrawn. Either standing or sitting, hold the water for a period of five to ten
minutes in order to liquefy the stools. Next, sit on the
toilet and release this injected liquid along with all the
matter that has dissolved into it.

Unlike the rectal douche, this procedure should be
performed only once at a time. Once is enough to evac-
uate sufficient wastes to bring the patient relief.

Summary

*Emptying the intestines is sometimes necessary during
a fever in order to reduce the quantity of wastes the
fever needs to burn.*

10

Adjusting Treatments according to Individual Needs

We have now looked at all the basic rules for applying the treatments offered by hydrotherapy, diet, and so forth. They have been presented in a broad manner and consequently offer only general instructions. Every patient presents a unique case; treatments must be adjusted to meet each patient's individual needs and every particular situation that may occur during the evolution of the fever. This is essential for gaining the greatest benefit from the various techniques available to us.

Hippocrates, the father of medicine, emphasized early on the necessity of being flexible and adapting treatments: "Often indeed medicine must do one thing at one time, and the next moment do the contrary. . . . When a severe diet causes harm, it should be replaced by a nourishing diet and, in this spirit, changed fairly frequently, with either this thing or that."

When a treatment procedure, for example, the application of cold water to reduce a fever, does not produce the desired effect and actually seems responsible for having negative ones, it is not enough to simply stop and do nothing. To the contrary, you now must apply an opposite treatment plan, which, in this case, would be to apply heat to the patient.

Like the balance of scales, health is an unstable equilibrium that requires constant restoration. There is a balance between the energy the body takes in and the energy it expends, between activity and rest, between the production and elimination of toxins, the production and loss of heat, and so forth. When the scales are tipped too far to one side, pressure must be exerted on the opposite side to restore an even balance.

In health care it is sometimes necessary to work one way, then another, then return to the first way, in order to keep organ function as close as possible to a position of ideal balance. To achieve this, it is essential to establish a patient chart. On this chart you will write all the important information concerning the progress of the patient's condition. In this way, you will be perfectly equipped to follow the fever's progression and intervene with appropriate corrective measures.

THE PATIENT CHART

Over the course of any illness numerous changes will be constantly occurring—changes in temperature, changes in symptoms, changes in the patient's overall condition. It is generally impossible to hold in your memory the precise moments such changes occurred. These details tend to quickly fall into oblivion, people become confused about the sequence of events after the fact—hence the need to write them down while they are still fresh.

A chart should be filled out for each day of the illness, with the date recorded. Each chart consists of three columns, allowing a record to be kept of what is ingested, general observations on the patient's condition and symptoms, and body temperature. Patient chart samples have been provided in this book's appendix.

Food and Beverages
This column should list all food and beverages the patient consumed on a given day of his illness. Record the kinds of foods eaten (vegetable, fruit, grain, dairy product, and so on) as well as the quantities of each— whether they were large or small. If the patient indulges in them, midmorning and midafternoon snacks should also be recorded.

During the stage of the fever when the patient is not eating anything, the corresponding parts of the chart should simply be left empty. This will allow you to see at a glance how long it has been since the patient ingested solid foods, when food was introduced back into his diet, the effect it had, and so forth.

All beverages should also be noted, even water. For example, 1 quart of water, 2 cups of lime-blossom tea, and so forth.

Observations on the Patient's Overall Condition and the Progress of Local Symptoms

Here you will note fluctuations in the patient's energy level, when the patient felt good or not, as well as the appearance, progression, and disappearance of all local symptoms (coughs, skin rashes and other outbreaks, pains, headaches, and so on). With respect to eliminations, it is good to write down the times when there were large bouts of perspiration and when stools were evacuated. It is also important to note those times when the patient got up to move around a little and when any hydrotherapy applications took place.

These observations should be recorded on the part of the chart relating to the time of day they took place: morning, afternoon, or night. This will make it easier to establish the cause and effect relationship in the sequence of events.

The Patient's Temperature

To get reliable temperature readings, it is important to always use the same thermometer in the same location (such as the armpit). As a general rule, temperature should be taken three times a day: in the morning on waking, in the afternoon around two o'clock, and in the evening between seven and eight o'clock. This last reading will be the most instructive as temperatures tend to rise during the evening. The absence of fever or a sharp drop in its temperature at that time indicates a good prognosis.

Summary

All methods for controlling fever (such as hydrotherapy and diet) should be adapted to each patient and each particular situation that appears over the course of the fever. Use of a patient chart is essential for accurately adapting treatments.

11

Complementary Care

There are a number of natural remedies that can be useful complements to the treatment methods recommended in the preceding chapters. These complementary options can be divided into two groups: The first consists of medicinal plants that will reduce the temperature of the fever. They are used only when the fever is too high or is lasting for too long despite the other treatments being administered to reduce the temperature. The second group consists of natural remedies that strengthen the body's defenses.

ANTIPYRETIC MEDICINAL PLANTS

The febrifuge properties of certain medicinal plants were discovered empirically and have been used for generations. In many cases, modern medicine has only confirmed what our ancestors already knew.

After all that I've said in this book about the benefits of fever, I am obviously not doing a complete about face here and recommending these plants be used to stop a fever. The fact that these are natural remedies rather than pharmaceutical preparations changes nothing in the basic equation. Any substance or method that cuts short a fever is cutting off the body's natural defenses at the same time, something that should be avoided as much as possible.

The reason I am devoting a section of the book to these remedies is that their use can be justified for very high fevers and those fevers that are lasting too long. In either of these cases, the effort demanded of the body can be too great and can endanger the patient. Antipyretic or febrifuge medicinal plants that can lower the temperature of a fever without suppressing it completely provide physical relief while allowing the body to continue fighting at a more manageable rhythm.

The first two plants presented below contain salicylic acid, a substance that acts on the center that is responsible for the body's heat management. Its febrifuge action, which impels the body to lower its overall temperature, is accompanied by a sudorific effect, which means it has the power to increase perspiration. The flavor and odor of this substance is quite unique, which you will discover if you drink a tea brewed from these plants. Its taste is, in fact, quite similar to that of aspirin. The active ingredient in aspirin is chemically very similar to salicylic acid, and aspirin was actually produced following the study of these plants.

White Willow (Salix alba)

White Willow is a small tree with silvery leaves that grows in damp places. Its active substances reside in its bark.

Decoction: To prepare a decoction, place ¾ ounce of crushed, dried bark in 1 quart of boiling water. Boil for five minutes and let steep for an additional ten minutes. Drink 2 or 3 cups a day.

Tablets or capsules: Follow manufacturer's instructions.

Meadowsweet (Spiraea ulmaria)

The flowering tops and leaves of this tall, elegant plant have long been used for their febrifuge effects. The plant grows in damp fields. It is the ancestor of the modern aspirin.

Infusion: To prepare an infusion, use 1 teaspoon of dried leaves and flowers per cup of boiling water. Let this steep for ten minutes. Drink 3 to 5 cups a day.

Tablets or capsules: Follow manufacturer's instructions.

The plants that follow are well known and have a pleasant taste. Their febrifuge effect comes from the fact that they all induce perspiration. By inducing the body to sweat copiously, they facilitate the elimination of toxins.

Black Elderberry *(Sambucus nigra)*

This tree produces clusters of small round berries that are a deep violet color. It is the flowers, though, that have been used since antiquity for their sudorific properties.

Infusion: To prepare an infusion, add a handful (about 1½ ounces) of dried flowers to 1 quart of boiling water. Let this steep for ten minutes. Drink 3 to 6 cups a day.

Linden *(or Common Lime)* *(*Tilia europaea*)*

Valued for their aromatic flavor, the flowers of the linden (or lime blossoms) help induce perspiration. This is why they are recommended for people suffering from fever as well as people in good health seeking a refreshing effect on a hot day.

Infusion: To prepare an infusion, add about 1 ounce of flowers to 1 quart of boiling water. Let steep for ten minutes. Drink 3 to 6 cups a day.

Roman or Garden Chamomile
(Anthemis nobilis)

This plant, which is primarily known for its use in relieving digestive disorders, is also a sudorific and a febrifuge.

Infusion: To prepare an infusion, add ¾ ounce of dried flowers to 1 quart of boiling water. Let steep for ten minutes. Drink 2 or 3 cups a day.

Eucalyptus (or Tasmanian bluegum)
(Eucalyptus globulus)

The reputation enjoyed by the eucalyptus tree for its prowess at lowering fever is confirmed by its folk name, "fever tree." Eucalyptus leaves have active properties that are both sudorific and disinfectant.

Infusion: To prepare an infusion, add about 1 ounce of dried leaves to 1 quart of boiling water. Let steep for fifteen minutes. Drink 3 to 5 cups a day.

REMEDIES TO STIMULATE THE BODY'S DEFENSE SYSTEM

All humans have a defense system at their disposal to confront whatever dangers threaten them. But all defense systems are not equal in strength. The effectiveness of the immune system is more or less dependent on the basic physiological forces received at birth, though its abilities can also vary over time. The immune system can also be diminished by fatigue, stress, poor nutrition, and the body's accumulation of toxins and poisons.

The body is therefore not always up to the task of properly protecting itself. It is sometimes necessary, depending on the case, to strengthen and stimulate, or reawaken, the body's defense mechanisms. There are a host of various remedies that make this stimulation of the immune system possible. In this section of the book, we will look at a few of the most effective ones.

Echinacea

Echinacea angustifolia, a member of the Asteraceae family, is a native of the North American prairies. It was used often and with great success by Native Americans to treat all kinds of ailments, and it plays a very helpful role in fevers.

It has an exceptional ability to stimulate the body's defense system by, among other things, producing white blood cells (macrophages) that attack and destroy the germs and poisons in the body's biological terrain. Echinacea also stimulates perspiration, which helps rid the body of these toxins. Furthermore, it reduces cellular exposure to infection and has an antibiotic effect against certain pathogenic germs. For all these reasons, echinacea is a major remedy for supporting the body's fight against disease.

The root of the plant is the primary part that is used. It is prepared in the form of an easy to use tincture.

Several small doses repeated throughout the day have a better effect than larger doses taken less frequently.

Dosage: Take 10 to 20 drops of the tincture, five to six times a day, with a little water.

Vitamin C

Vitamin C is a useful substance for maintaining the body's general functioning, but when taken at higher doses it has amazing therapeutic virtues that have been confirmed by modern studies.

Vitamin C stimulates the body's defenses by making white blood cells and antibodies more effective in their battle against infection. It kills microbes and viruses, and neutralizes numerous poisons. Because it stimulates the overall health of the body, vitamin C is always recommended for the additional support it provides the struggling body during a fever. During a fever the body needs more than 1,000 mg of vitamin C a day. According to some authors, the daily amount ingested can even be equal to several grams. The natural vitamin C supplements available in the market generally have a fairly low dosage (50 to 100 mg), but there are some preparations that are 500 to 1,000 mg. These are the ones you should obviously use to obtain effective therapeutic results.

Dosage: Take 1 to 3 grams a day, broken up into several doses over the course of the day.

Magnesium Chloride

The effectiveness of the white blood cells that defend the body against microbial infections and poisoning depends on the composition of the surrounding environment. If the amount of an essential substance falls below its normal levels, the white blood cells will work less well, whereas when the levels of this substance are elevated, their defensive capabilities are substantially increased.

Magnesium chloride is one of these substances on which the effectiveness of the immune system depends. Diseased bodies generally display a deficiency in this essential substance. Taking magnesium chloride as a supplement addresses this deficiency and stimulates the body's defenses.

The use of magnesium chloride is quite simple. Packets can often be found in natural health stores and supermarkets. Empty the packet into a glass of water, and the remedy is ready to be imbibed. One dose corresponds to 125 cc of solution, thus in the general neighborhood of an ordinary drinking glass.

Dosage: At the first signs of fever, drink 1 glass at three-hour intervals, until 3 glasses have been drunk. For the next two days, drink 1 glass every six hours. After the two days, reduce to 2 glasses a day for three days, then 1 glass a day for a week.

Magnesium chloride has a distinctive flavor that can be avoided by drinking it down in one gulp rather than sipping it. It can also have a laxative effect on some people. This is only temporary and can be toned down by lowering the dose. Keep in mind, though, that this is not a negative reaction. Emptying the intestines is helping the body rid itself of the toxins that are clogging its systems.

Magnesium chloride is also available in tablet and liquid form. Follow the manufacturer's dosage guidelines.

Trace Elements

Trace elements are minerals that are present in very small amounts in foods. They contribute to the sound and proper functioning of the body. Every trace element stimulates one or more organic functions or biochemical reactions. A deficiency in a trace element will cause reduced capacity of the function dependent on it. This reduction in the physiological function will grow worse as long as the body receives no intake of this trace element.

Trace elements are like tiny sparks that keep the body's motor running. They are therefore even more valuable when the body becomes exhausted in its struggle, as can be the case during a fever, and requires assistance to perform all its functions properly.

The trace elements of copper, gold, and silver are most apt to stimulate the exhausted defenses of the body. There are liquid preparations available commercially that contain all three of these trace elements. To encourage maximum absorption, it is best to take the remedy on an empty stomach and hold it beneath your tongue for a minute before swallowing. This part of the mouth has a vast number of blood vessels, which permits the active properties of these elements to enter the bloodstream rapidly.

Dosage: One dose is generally around 30 drops of the preparation* and should be taken once or twice a day before eating.

Summary

The use of natural sweat-inducing and immune-strengthening remedies can enhance the body's own efforts to restore health.

---

*Always follow manufacturer's instructions to account for different preparation strengths.

12

Creating an Artificial Fever

Once you understand the importance of a healthy cellular environment and the power of fever in burning away toxins and renewing this biological terrain, you cannot help but admire the wisdom of nature in creating fever to help us recover our health. Invading germs as well as ingested poisons that have accumulated over time from unhealthy lifestyle choices can all be eliminated in a relatively short time by one simple, but intense process: fever.

Everyone knows that "an ounce of prevention is worth a pound of cure." The later a treatment is started, the greater the deterioration of the body's biological terrain will be. By using preventive measures to avoid deterioration of the terrain in the first place, you can prevent disease from getting a foothold. This is why, rather than forcing the body to unleash a fever, it is far better to avoid reaching this state of decline by cleansing the cellular terrain in advance, just like a fever would.

But is it possible to create an artificial fever? This is a question that has been a subject of concern to health care practitioners for some time now. Attention to this question has fortunately led to the discovery of simple, natural methods for inducing fever, methods that can be used whenever there is a need to take this kind of preventive measure.

There are two methods that are particularly effective in creating fever: hyperthermal baths and sustained physical exercise. With the baths the heat is brought to the body from the outside, while with physical exercise the body produces the heat itself. The first procedure is therefore more passive and the second more active, but both are equally valid and effective. The main distinction is that they are best suited for people whose physical capabilities are different.

In both methods, the heat intensifies blood circulation, oxygenation of tissues, combustion of wastes, cellular exchanges, elimination of toxins, and the body's defenses, in the same way a fever does. Also in both cases, the core temperature no longer remains confined to the interior of the body but is spread until it reaches the skin surface, ensuring that the entire body benefits from the healthy effects of the fever.

While these techniques make it possible to produce a strong fever, it will only be a temporary condition, lasting for one or two hours rather than the several days that a natural fever can continue. A complete, definitive result will therefore not occur with just one treatment. The chosen method should be repeated several times a week in order to achieve the desired regeneration of the body's biological terrain.

Let's now take a look at how to receive the maximum benefits from these techniques while respecting our physiological boundaries. This does not involve, for example, filling your bathtub with the hottest water possible or exercising until you have reached a state of complete exhaustion. There are very logical and precise boundaries that should govern the application of these treatments.

HYPERTHERMAL BATHS

As their name indicates, *hyperthermal baths* are very hot baths. But the sensation of heat is a subjective matter, which is why there is no precise temperature that the water must reach. Everyone needs to discover their own ideal temperature.

This works in the following way: Get into a bathtub with several inches of water heated to body temperature, 98.6°F. Next, continue raising the temperature of the bath gradually by adding hotter water until you reach your tolerance threshold, which would be just before the point at which you can no longer stand the heat. Fill the bathtub with enough water to cover your entire body, except your head, of course.

Despite its high temperature, the bath should not be so hot that you cannot tolerate the heat; you should feel at ease. The goal is not to try to stand the highest heat possible but to find the temperature that will allow you to spend half an hour in the bath comfortably. Depending on your personal threshold, the temperature should be in the neighborhood of 102°F to 108°F.

The purpose of the hyperthermal bath is to bring a large amount of heat to the body. If you have a low heat threshold, this objective can still be attained by spending a longer time in water that is not quite so hot. Since the bath will have a tendency to lose heat during this time span, do not hesitate to add more hot water to it as needed. In anticipation of these necessary additions, it is a good idea to not fill the bathtub completely at the onset. The more water in the bathtub, and the lower its temperature, the harder it will be to reheat.

On the other end of the spectrum, it is important to stress that you should not suddenly immerse yourself in extremely hot water, even if it is at a temperature you can tolerate. In fact, the body's initial defensive reaction to this sudden assault will be to close the pores of the skin, which would partially negate the desired effect.

It is imperative to allow the body to get used to hyperthermal baths. There should be no hesitation about increasing both the temperature and duration of these baths very gradually over a period of several weeks before reaching their maximum potential. As a precautionary measure, and to avoid head congestion, you can keep a cold washcloth on your forehead during the bath.

Depending on your personal constitution and vitality, a hyperthermal bath may be taken every two or three days for a period of several months, or every day for one or two weeks.

Once finished bathing, gently climb out of the tub and lie down for a half hour or more wrapped in a terrycloth towel and a blanket. This extended period of rest allows the body to complete sweating and restore its balance. Because the bath was at least half an hour in duration, a great deal of heat collected in the body. The artificially induced fever will not stop as soon as you get out of the bath; it continues working, gradually subsiding. You will therefore continue to perspire heavily for a good part of this rest period.

Because the power of hyperthermal baths is their high heat, it is not necessary to add any special preparation to the water, for example, a mixture of medicinal herbs. However, there is also no reason not to do so. In addition, teas with sweat-inducing ingredients such as lime and elder blossoms can be drunk, piping hot, before and after the bath.

The artificial fever that results from immersing the body in hot water can easily be verified by taking an oral temperature reading. This artificial fever shares the same properties as a naturally occurring fever. Combustions intensify and the wastes that are scattered throughout the body, some lodged deep within the tissue, are broken down and eliminated.

In a hyperthermal bath, the body feels as if it is under attack from the heat of the water and that its thermal equilibrium is threatened. This prompts it to react and defend itself in three different ways, all of which are similar to the reactions that take place during a natural fever.

1. The vessels dilate because the body is attempting to open all its pathways to the outside to their maximum extent in order to retain the least amount of heat possible. This vessel dilation occurs most prominently at the level of the capillaries, which play a major role in the irrigation of the body's deepest tissues.

   When the capillaries dilate, the surface area of the exchange between the cellular tissues and the bloodstream increases, thereby permitting the extraction and elimination of toxins lodged in the cells. Circulation can be reestablished in the poorly irrigated regions of the body, which had become like swamps or deserts because of the surcharge of toxins and the poor functioning of the capillaries.

Overburdened capillaries are like dams on the exit paths for these deep toxins. By dilating these small blood vessels, the hyperthermal bath opens an exit door for embedded, non-circulating toxins and activates the process of cellular exchange. This makes it possible for toxins to rise from the deepest levels and enter the bloodstream where they will be carried to an excretory organ and eliminated from the body.

2. Blood circulation accelerates, which, by preventing the blood from remaining in contact with the heat source for too long, cools the overheated tissues with fresh infusions of cooler blood. Evidence of this physiological acceleration can be heard in the stronger and more rapid heartbeat. The blood, by increasing its speed of circulation, sweeps away wastes that have built up on the vessel walls and transports them to the excretory organs to be eliminated from the body. Furthermore, the increase in the speed of the blood flow causes an acceleration of lymphatic circulation.

3. The skin perspires, reducing heat through the evaporation of sweat while excreting numerous toxins from the body, as would be the case with a naturally occurring fever.

Hyperthermal baths have a much more powerful effect than most people imagine. In fact, if you neglect to follow the gradual progression recommended earlier, you can trigger a massive elimination of deeply embedded toxins, or what is known as a cleansing crisis. When these embedded toxins are brought suddenly into the bloodstream and combined with the toxins already circulating there, they can completely overwhelm the eliminatory capacities of the excretory organs. Unpleasant side effects such as headaches and nausea can result. These disagreeable reactions can be avoided by gradually building up to the highest tolerable heat threshold.

Without reaching the extremes of a cleansing, or healing, crisis, you can still see the purifying effects of these baths in the urine, which should be darker and more charged with wastes, and in the tear ducts, which will secrete more "sand" and so forth.

There are some criticisms that have been levied against hyperthermal baths, such as:

They might be bad for the heart. It is true that during a hyperthermal bath the heart is forced to work harder. But we should not overlook the fact that the heart is a muscle and like all muscles it can tolerate more substantial efforts, as long as it becomes *gradually* accustomed to taking on a greater workload. People with known heart conditions should ask their physician before taking hyperthermal baths.

They could possibly be harmful for those afflicted with varicose veins. In theory, no, quite the contrary: by encouraging circulation, varicose veins should fade away. But in practice, this is not always the case. The patient can then try bathing with her legs out of the water and showering her legs with very cold water after getting out of the tub to prevent the blood from descending into the lower limbs. An individual suffering from this condition could also try to remain lying down with her legs elevated. If the varicose veins dilate despite these precautions, then it will be necessary for the patient to stop taking hyperthermal baths.

SUSTAINED PHYSICAL EXERCISE

Sustained physical exercise is the second practice capable of creating an artificial fever. In fact, all physical effort produces heat as it causes the muscles to contract, the heart to beat faster, blood circulation to accelerate, and the lungs to breathe more deeply. The longer the effort continues, the greater the tendency for heat to collect and, as a consequence, the overall body temperature to rise. This places the individual in a state of artificial fever that burns away the toxins that have collected in the biological terrain. During a protracted, intense physical effort, the body temperature can climb as high as 104°F, which is at the line between a high and very high fever.

While physical exercise causes the combustion of the body's energetic reserves, it is also breaking down wastes. In fact, intense physical effort necessarily engenders a much more intense level of oxygenation, which provides better oxidation on the cellular level—oxidation also breaks down wastes and toxins.

When a normally sedentary person makes a physical effort, exhaustion appears quite soon. The body quickly becomes overwhelmed by the oxidations being spurred on by this increased activity. With training, exhaustion will intervene with less frequency and the body will become increasingly accustomed to oxidizing at deeper and deeper levels.

The additional cellular oxygenation and increased energy needs caused by sustained physical exercise burn away the body's wastes all the way down to the cellular level. The toxins that are more or less embedded in the tissues will be broken down on the spot.

To obtain these results, the physical exercise should be comparable to the effort required for sports such as cycling, long distance running, cross country skiing, and so on. For those who have the strength necessary to perform activities like these, pursuing them for a period of one or two hours makes it possible to create an artificial fever. Repeated on a regular basis, this will contribute greatly to restoring the integrity of the internal cellular environment.

The length of the exercise session should obviously be in accord with the physiological capacities of the individual. Overexerting yourself in an effort to obtain better results is a bad gamble. The high production of toxins and exhaustion of the body this will cause wipes out the benefits that the artificial fever could otherwise have provided.

One way to reduce the muscular effort required while maintaining the strong heating effect of the body is to perform gentler forms of exercise such as walking, gardening, a short bike ride, gymnastics, and so forth on a hot summer day so that the heat produced by the body will be added to that supplied by the ambient air. During other seasons performing these milder activities while wearing warm clothing will achieve a similar effect. This allows the exercise to be much milder while still attaining the heat required to create a fever.

The regular practice of artificially produced fevers will cleanse the depths of the biological terrain, which in turn will bring about health and vitality and prevent the return of illness.

Summary

Creating an artificial fever, through hyperthermal baths or sustained physical exercise, provides a means for forestalling illnesses by ridding the biological terrain of toxins, just as a natural fever would.

Patient Chart

Instructions for filling out a patient chart are provided in chapter 10 (see pages 105–7).

DATE: _____

Food and Beverages	Observations	Temperature
Morning	Morning	Morning
Noon	Afternoon	2 p.m.
Evening	Night	Evening

DATE: _____

Food and Beverages	Observations	Temperature
Morning	Morning	Morning
Noon	Afternoon	2 p.m.
Evening	Night	Evening

DATE: _____

Food and Beverages	Observations	Temperature
Morning	Morning	Morning
Noon	Afternoon	2 p.m.
Evening	Night	Evening

Index